Food Macros Made Easy

Macros for Beginners. A guide to understanding macros nutrition and counting macros. Learn to tailor a macro diet for beginners, including adjusting macros for weight loss.

By: Amelia Evans

Abstract

In 'Food Macros Made Easy,' we embark on a transformative journey into the world of nutrition science made simple. This comprehensive guide breaks down complex nutritional concepts into digestible, practical knowledge that you can immediately apply to your daily life. Whether you're looking to optimize your athletic performance, manage your weight, or learn how to fuel your body more effectively, this book provides the foundational knowledge and practical tools you need to succeed. Through clear explanations, real-world examples, and flexible strategies, you'll learn how to master macro-nutrition while maintaining an enjoyable and sustainable relationship with food.

Table of Contents

Introduction

Have you ever stood in your kitchen, staring at your meal, wondering if you're making the right food choices? I've been there, and so have countless others on their nutrition journey. Like many of you, I once believed that healthy eating meant restrictive diets and complicated calculations. That was until I discovered the transformative power of understanding macronutrients—the fundamental building blocks that fuel our bodies and shape our health.

When I first began exploring nutrition, I was overwhelmed by conflicting information and rigid rules. It wasn't until I started breaking down my meals into their basic components—proteins, carbohydrates, and fats—that nutrition finally started making sense. This simple shift in perspective changed everything, not just for me, but for the countless individuals I've had the privilege of guiding on their wellness journeys.

In this book, we'll demystify macro-nutrition and transform it from a complex science into practical, everyday wisdom. You'll learn why understanding macronutrients is like learning the alphabet before writing a story - it gives you the fundamental tools to create a nutrition plan that works for your unique body and lifestyle. Whether you're an athlete looking to optimize performance, someone seeking sustainable weight management, or simply wanting to improve your overall health, this guide will show you how to make macro-nutrition work for you.

You won't find rigid meal plans or one-size-fits-all solutions here. Instead, we'll explore flexible strategies that adapt to your life, practical tools for tracking without becoming obsessed, and real-world solutions for maintaining a balanced diet in any situation. Through personal stories, useful examples, and evidence-based insights, I'll demonstrate how understanding macros can transform your relationship with food, helping you achieve your health and fitness goals.

What sets this guide apart is its focus on sustainability and personalization. We'll discuss how to adapt macro-nutrition principles to different body types, lifestyles, and goals. You'll learn how to navigate restaurants, social events, and busy schedules while maintaining your nutrition targets. Most importantly, you'll learn how to transform macro awareness into lasting habits that support your well-being without dominating your life.

As we begin this journey together, remember that mastering macro-nutrition isn't about achieving perfection - it's about gaining the knowledge and tools to make informed choices that support your health goals. Whether you're new to nutrition or looking to refine your existing knowledge, this book will serve as your practical guide to understanding and implementing macro-nutrition principles in your daily life.

Let's move beyond the confusion of fad diets and rigid rules. It's time to discover how understanding and balancing macronutrients can lead to sustainable, enjoyable, and adequate nutrition that transforms not only your body but also your entire approach to healthy living. Welcome to your journey of macro mastery - let's begin.

Chapter 1

———————⌃———————

Understanding Macros:
The Building Blocks of Nutrition

Every time you sit down for a meal, you're not just eating food - you're fueling your body with three essential macronutrients that serve as the foundation of human nutrition. Understanding these macronutrients—proteins, carbohydrates, and fats—is like learning the alphabet before writing a story; they're the basic building blocks that, when properly balanced, create the narrative of your health and wellness journey. Just as the letters combine to form words that convey meaning, these macronutrients work together to fuel our bodies, support our health, and help us achieve our wellness goals. Like many readers starting their nutrition journey, my path to understanding macronutrients began with confusion and misconceptions.

When I first started my journey into nutrition, I was overwhelmed by conflicting information about what to eat. Like many of my clients, I used to believe that all fats were bad and protein was only for bodybuilders. One day, while preparing lunch for my family, I decided to analyze our typical meal: a sandwich with whole-grain bread, turkey, avocado, and vegetables. This simple exercise became my 'aha' moment. I realized that this everyday meal contained all three macronutrients in action: the bread provided carbohydrates for energy, the turkey delivered essential protein for muscle maintenance, and the avocado offered healthy fats for nutrient absorption and brain health. This revelation transformed my view of food, not as 'good' or 'bad,' but as different building blocks working together. This new perspective not only changed my approach to nutrition but also helped me develop a more balanced relationship with food.

Now, when I teach macro-nutrition to others, I often use this sandwich analogy to demonstrate how these nutrients work together in harmony, making the complex world of nutrition more approachable and understandable. Throughout this chapter, we'll break down the role of each macronutrient in your body, exploring how they function individually and collectively to support your health and wellness goals. You'll discover that understanding macronutrients isn't about memorizing complex biochemistry - it's about recognizing the powerful building blocks that make up your daily meals.

Just as a house needs a solid foundation, your nutrition journey begins with understanding these fundamental components. We'll explore practical ways to identify these macronutrients in everyday foods, learn how to balance them effectively, and discover how they contribute to your overall health and energy levels. Whether your goal is weight management, improved athletic performance, or simply better health, mastering these basics will empower you to make informed choices about your nutrition.

As we delve deeper into each macronutrient, you'll gain confidence in recognizing their sources and understanding their importance in your daily diet. This knowledge will serve as the cornerstone for the more advanced concepts we'll explore in later chapters, building a comprehensive understanding of nutrition that will serve you well on your wellness journey.

The Three Macronutrients: Proteins, Carbohydrates, and Fats Explained

Let's dive into the three macronutrients that form the foundation of our nutrition - think of them as the primary colors that, when appropriately combined, create a masterpiece of health and wellness. Each plays a vital and unique role in maintaining the optimal functioning of our bodies.

First, let's meet protein, often referred to as the body's building block. Imagine your body as a constantly renovating house - protein provides the materials needed for repairs, maintenance, and new construction. It's essential for building and maintaining muscle tissue, supporting immune function, and creating necessary enzymes and hormones. You'll find protein in foods like eggs, lean meats, fish, legumes, and dairy products. A palm-sized portion of protein-rich food typically contains about 20-30 grams of protein, making it easy to accurately estimate your portion size.

Next up are carbohydrates, your body's preferred energy source. Think of carbohydrates as your body's power plant - they provide the fuel needed for everything from essential bodily functions to intense physical activity. They come in two primary forms: complex carbohydrates found in whole grains, vegetables, and legumes, which provide sustained energy; and simple carbohydrates found in fruits and processed foods, which offer quick energy. Your cupped hand can serve as a useful measuring tool for carbohydrate portions, typically holding about 30-40 grams of carbohydrates.

Lastly, we have fats, which have been unfairly demonized in the past but are crucial for health. Fats are like the oil in your car's engine - essential for smooth operation and proper maintenance. They help absorb vital nutrients, support brain health, and maintain cell structures. Healthy fats can be found in foods like avocados, nuts, olive oil, and fatty fish. Your thumb can serve as a helpful guide for fat portions, with the size of your thumb tip representing approximately 7-9 grams of fat.

The beauty of these macronutrients lies in their synergy. Just as a well-composed photograph requires the right balance of elements, your body performs optimally when these macronutrients work in harmony. For example, when you eat an apple with almond butter, the fat from the nuts helps slow down the absorption of the fruit's carbohydrates, providing more sustained energy. Similarly, consuming carbohydrates with protein after exercise helps support muscle recovery more effectively than either nutrient alone.

Understanding how to balance these macronutrients doesn't require complex calculations or strict rules. Start by visualizing your plate: aim for a palm-sized portion of protein, a cupped hand of carbohydrates, and a thumb-sized portion of healthy fats at each main meal. This straightforward approach offers a practical foundation that you can tailor to your individual needs and goals.

Remember, while these proportions provide a helpful starting point, your individual needs may vary depending on factors such as age, activity level, and specific health goals. Some people thrive on higher carbohydrate intakes, while others feel better with a higher intake of protein or fat. The key is learning to listen to your body while maintaining awareness of these basic building blocks.

As we progress through this book, we'll explore how to fine-tune these ratios for your specific needs and learn practical strategies for incorporating them into your daily meals. For now, focus on identifying these macronutrients in your current diet and noting how different combinations affect your overall well-being. This awareness will serve as the foundation for the more detailed strategies we'll discuss in later chapters.

Energy Balance: How Macros Fuel Your Body

Think of your body as a sophisticated hybrid car that can run on multiple fuel sources. Just as a hybrid vehicle can switch between electricity and gasoline, your body expertly utilizes different macronutrients for energy based on your activities and needs. Understanding this energy balance is crucial for optimizing your nutrition and achieving your health goals.

I learned this lesson firsthand during my transition from a desk job to becoming a more active nutrition and wellness coach. Initially, I couldn't understand why I felt constantly drained despite eating what I thought was a healthy diet. The problem wasn't the quality of my food - it was the balance of my energy sources. I was consuming too few carbohydrates for my new activity level, leaving my body struggling to maintain consistent energy throughout the day.

Energy balance is fundamentally about matching your energy input (the food you eat) with your energy output, which includes your daily activities and exercise. Each macronutrient contributes differently to this energy equation. Carbohydrates are like your body's premium gasoline - they're the preferred and most efficient energy source for most activities, especially high-intensity exercise. Proteins serve as both building materials and a backup energy source, while fats are like your body's deep energy reserves, perfect for sustained, lower-intensity activities.

Your body is remarkably adaptable in its use of these different energy sources. During a typical day, you naturally cycle through various fuel sources. When you wake up, your body primarily relies on stored fat for energy. During exercise, it preferentially uses carbohydrates for quick energy. During extended periods without food, it can convert protein and fat into usable forms of energy. This metabolic flexibility is key to maintaining stable energy levels throughout the day.

To visualize this energy balance, imagine your daily energy needs as a bank account. Your macronutrient intake represents deposits, while your activities are withdrawals. Just as you wouldn't want to overdraw your bank account, you need to ensure your energy intake matches your needs. However, this doesn't mean you need to count every calorie meticulously. Instead, focus on understanding how different combinations of macronutrients affect your energy levels.

For example, a breakfast high in protein and healthy fats, like eggs with avocado, provides sustained energy throughout the morning. A lunch rich in complex carbohydrates and protein, such as quinoa with grilled chicken and vegetables, helps maintain energy levels throughout the afternoon.

On active days, you may increase your carbohydrate intake to support higher energy demands. Conversely, on less active days, you may reduce carbohydrate intake and increase protein and fat intake.

The key to mastering energy balance lies in recognizing your body's signals. When your macro balance is correct, you'll experience consistent energy levels, a stable mood, and better recovery from exercise. When it's off, you might notice energy crashes, increased hunger, or poor exercise performance. These signals are your body's way of communicating its energy needs.

One of my clients, Sarah, discovered this through her own experience. As a busy professional who enjoyed morning workouts, she struggled with mid-afternoon energy crashes. By adjusting her macro balance to include more complex carbohydrates around her workouts and ensuring adequate protein throughout the day, she found her energy levels stabilized. This simple adjustment in her macro timing made a significant difference in her daily performance.

Remember that energy balance isn't about achieving perfect ratios every day. It's about understanding how different macronutrients fuel your body and learning to adjust them based on your activities and goals. On some days, you may need more carbohydrates for high-energy activities, while on other days, you may require more fats and proteins for sustained, steady energy. The flexibility to adjust your macro intake according to your changing needs is what makes this approach sustainable in the long term.

As we continue through this book, you'll learn more specific strategies for adjusting your macro balance to support different goals and activities. For now, start paying attention to how different macro combinations affect your energy levels throughout the day. This awareness will become invaluable as you develop your approach to macro nutrition.

Protein: The Building Blocks of Life

When I first began studying nutrition, I was fascinated by how a single macronutrient could play such a crucial role in our body. Protein truly is the master builder of our physical form, serving as the foundation for everything from our muscles and bones to our skin and immune system. Like skilled construction workers on a building site, proteins are constantly at work, repairing, maintaining, and creating new structures throughout our bodies.

Think of protein as the versatile building blocks in a massive LEGO set - each piece can be assembled and reassembled in countless ways to create different structures your body needs. These building blocks, known as amino acids, combine in various patterns to form everything from muscle tissue to essential enzymes and hormones. Your body can produce some of these amino acids on its own, but nine essential amino acids must come from your diet, making protein intake a vital part of your daily nutrition.

I recall working with a client named Mark, who was struggling to understand why his recovery from workouts was so slow, despite his dedicated exercise routine. When we analyzed his diet, we found that his protein intake was significantly below what his active lifestyle required. By gradually increasing his protein intake through strategic meal planning, incorporating foods such as lean meats, eggs, legumes, and dairy products, his recovery improved significantly. This transformation highlighted a crucial lesson: adequate protein isn't just for bodybuilders - it's essential for everyone, from office workers to athletes.

The beauty of protein lies in its diverse roles in our body. Beyond building muscle, protein helps maintain healthy skin, hair, and nails, supports immune function, and aids in the production of enzymes that digest food and hormones that regulate various bodily functions. It's also beneficial for weight management, as protein tends to be more satiating than other macronutrients, helping you feel fuller for more extended periods.

Let's break down some practical guidelines for protein intake. A general starting point is consuming 0.8-1.0 grams of protein per kilogram of body weight for sedentary adults, with active individuals potentially needing more. However, rather than getting caught up in precise calculations, I teach my clients to use simple visual guides. A palm-sized portion of protein-rich food at each meal is a good target for most people. This might be a chicken breast, a piece of fish, a cup of lentils, or a serving of Greek yogurt.

Quality matters as much as quantity when it comes to protein. Complete proteins, which contain all the essential amino acids, can be found in animal sources such as meat, fish, eggs, and dairy products. Plant-based proteins, while sometimes incomplete individually, can be combined throughout the day to provide all necessary amino acids. For example, pairing rice with beans creates a complete protein profile.

Timing your protein intake throughout the day can also enhance its benefits. Rather than consuming most of your protein in one meal, aim to distribute it across your daily meals and snacks. This approach helps maintain a steady supply of amino acids for your body's ongoing repair and maintenance needs. For instance, starting your day with eggs or Greek yogurt, having a tuna sandwich at lunch, and including a serving of lean protein at dinner provides a good distribution pattern.

One common misconception I often encounter is that high protein intake is harmful to kidney function. While individuals with existing kidney disease may need to monitor their protein intake, research has consistently shown that healthy individuals can safely consume recommended amounts of protein without adverse effects. However, as with all aspects of nutrition, moderation and balance are key.

For those new to tracking protein intake, start by focusing on including a quality protein source at each main meal. Pay attention to how different amounts of protein affect your hunger levels, energy, and recovery from physical activity. This awareness will help you fine-tune your intake to match your individual needs and goals.

Remember, while protein is crucial, it's just one part of a balanced nutrition approach. In the following sections, we'll explore how to combine protein effectively with carbohydrates and fats to create meals that support your overall health and wellness goals. The key is finding a sustainable approach that works for your lifestyle while ensuring you're getting the protein your body needs to thrive.

Carbohydrates: Understanding Your Body's Primary Fuel Source

Carbohydrates often get a bad rap in popular diet culture. Still, they're your body's preferred source of energy - think of them as the premium fuel that keeps your engine running smoothly. I learned this lesson the hard way during my early days of nutrition coaching when I attempted a very low-carb diet while maintaining an active lifestyle. My energy plummeted, my workouts suffered, and I found myself struggling to focus during client sessions. This experience taught me a valuable lesson about the essential role carbohydrates play in our daily functioning.

Carbohydrates are like the power plants of our cellular energy system. When you eat carbohydrates, your body breaks them down into glucose, which serves as the primary fuel source for your brain, muscles, and other vital organs. Your brain alone uses about 20% of your body's glucose-derived energy, which explains why you might feel foggy or irritable when your carbohydrate intake is too low.

There are two main types of carbohydrates: simple and complex. Simple carbohydrates, found in foods like fruits, milk, and refined sugars, are quickly broken down and absorbed, providing rapid energy. Complex carbohydrates, found in whole grains, vegetables, and legumes, are digested more slowly, providing sustained energy release over time. Think of simple carbs as kindling that quickly ignites to start a fire, while complex carbs are like logs that burn slowly and steadily.

One of my clients, Lisa, came to me frustrated with her afternoon energy crashes. She had been skipping carbs at lunch in an attempt to lose weight, only to find herself reaching for sugary snacks by mid-afternoon. We adjusted her lunch to include complex carbohydrates, such as quinoa or sweet potatoes, paired with protein and healthy fats. The result? Stable energy levels throughout the afternoon and no more sugar cravings. This transformation highlighted how proper carbohydrate timing and selection can support sustained energy and better food choices.

Understanding portion sizes for carbohydrates doesn't require complicated calculations. A good starting point is using your cupped hand as a portion guide, which typically represents about 30-40 grams of carbohydrates; however, needs vary based on activity level and goals. For example, someone training for a marathon would need significantly more carbohydrates than someone with a sedentary lifestyle.

The quality of your carbohydrate choices matters as much as the quantity. Fiber-rich complex carbohydrates not only provide sustained energy but also support digestive health and help maintain stable blood sugar levels. Foods like oats, brown rice, quinoa, sweet potatoes, and legumes are excellent sources of complex carbohydrates. These foods are also rich in essential vitamins, minerals, and fiber, which contribute to overall health.

Timing your carbohydrate intake can significantly impact its effectiveness. For example, consuming carbohydrates before exercise can provide the energy needed for optimal performance, while consuming carbohydrates after exercise helps replenish energy stores and support recovery. I often recommend that my clients follow what I call the 'activity matching' principle, adjusting their carbohydrate intake based on their daily activity levels and timing.

A common concern I hear from clients is whether carbohydrates cause weight gain. The truth is that any macronutrient consumed more than your body's needs can contribute to weight gain. The key is finding the right balance for your activity level and goals. Some people thrive on a higher intake of carbohydrates, while others feel better with moderate amounts. The key is to select high-quality sources and adjust portions according to your individual needs.

For those new to managing their carbohydrate intake, start by focusing on quality rather than quantity. Replace refined carbohydrates with whole food sources, observe how different types of carbohydrates affect your energy levels, and pay attention to the timing. This awareness will help you develop an intuitive understanding of your body's carbohydrate needs.

Remember, carbohydrates aren't your enemy - they're a vital tool in your nutrition toolkit. The key is learning how to use them effectively to support your health and performance goals. As we continue through this book, you'll learn more specific strategies for incorporating carbohydrates into your meal planning and how to adjust your intake based on different activities and goals.

Healthy Fats: Essential Functions and Best Sources

For years, dietary fats were unfairly demonized in the nutrition community, but we now understand that they play essential roles in our health and well-being. Like the oil in a well-maintained machine, healthy fats keep our bodies running smoothly, supporting everything from brain function to hormone production. When I first began learning about nutrition, I was surprised to discover how many vital bodily processes rely on adequate fat intake.

I remember working with a client named Rachel who had been following an extremely low-fat diet in an attempt to lose weight. She complained of constant hunger, dry skin, and difficulty concentrating. When we gradually reintroduced healthy fats into her diet through foods like avocados, olive oil, and nuts, she experienced improved satiety, better skin health, and enhanced mental clarity. This transformation highlighted the crucial role that healthy fats play in our overall wellness.

Healthy fats serve multiple essential functions in our bodies. They help absorb fat-soluble vitamins (A, D, E, and K), maintain cell membrane structure, support brain health, and provide a concentrated source of energy. They're also crucial for hormone production and regulation, which affects everything from metabolism to mood. Think of healthy fats as the body's natural insulation system - they help maintain body temperature, protect organs, and store energy when needed most.

When it comes to choosing healthy fats, quality is just as important as quantity. There are several types of beneficial fats we should include in our diet:

- Monounsaturated fats found in olive oil, avocados, and nuts

- Omega-3 fatty acids present in fatty fish, flaxseeds, and chia seeds

- Some saturated fats from sources like coconut oil and grass-fed butter

A good starting point for portion control is using your thumb as a guide - the size of your thumb typically represents about 7-9 grams of fat, which is a reasonable serving size for oils and nut butters. For whole food sources like avocados or nuts, a small handful or quarter of an avocado provides a good portion of healthy fats.

Incorporating healthy fats into your daily meals doesn't have to be complicated. Start your day with eggs cooked in olive oil, add avocado to your lunch salad, and include a handful of nuts as an afternoon snack. For dinner, consider fatty fish like salmon or mackerel, which provide both protein and beneficial omega-3 fats. These simple additions can significantly enhance the nutritional value of your meals while also improving flavor and satisfaction.

One common concern I hear from clients is whether consuming fat will cause them to gain weight. The truth is, fats are more calorie-dense than other macronutrients, containing 9 calories per gram compared to 4 calories per gram for proteins and carbohydrates. However, when consumed in moderation as part of a balanced diet, healthy fats can support weight management by enhancing satiety and helping to stabilize blood sugar levels.

The key to incorporating healthy fats is finding the right balance for your individual needs. Some people thrive on a higher intake of fat, while others feel better with moderate amounts. Pay attention to how different fat sources and quantities affect your energy levels, satiety, and overall well-being. This awareness will help you determine your optimal fat intake.

Timing can also play a role in how we use dietary fats. Including some healthy fats with each meal can help slow digestion and provide sustained energy. For example, adding olive oil to your vegetables not only enhances flavor but also helps your body absorb fat-soluble nutrients more effectively. Similarly, including some nuts or seeds with your afternoon snack can help prevent energy crashes between meals.

For those new to tracking fat intake, start by focusing on incorporating one serving of healthy fats at each main meal. This might mean adding avocado to your breakfast, using olive oil-based dressing on your lunch salad, and cooking your dinner vegetables in coconut oil. As you become more comfortable, you can adjust portions based on your individual needs and goals.

Remember that while healthy fats are essential, they're just one piece of the nutrition puzzle. The key is finding a balanced approach that includes all macronutrients in proportions that work for your body and lifestyle. As we continue through this book, you'll learn more specific strategies for combining fats, proteins, and carbohydrates to create satisfying, nutritious meals that support your health goals. As we conclude this foundational chapter on macronutrients, let's reflect on how these essential building blocks—proteins, carbohydrates, and fats—work together to support our overall health and well-being. Like the simple sandwich example I shared at the beginning of this chapter, every meal is an opportunity to nourish your body with these vital nutrients in balance.

Through our exploration of each macronutrient, we've discovered how proteins serve as the body's construction crew, rebuilding and maintaining tissues while supporting immune function. We've learned that carbohydrates act as our primary energy source, fueling everything from brain function to physical activity. And we've rehabilitated the reputation of healthy fats, understanding their crucial role in hormone production, nutrient absorption, and brain health.

Remember that successful macro-nutrition isn't about perfect calculations or rigid rules - it's about understanding these fundamental components and learning to balance them in a way that works for your unique body and lifestyle. The hand-portion guidelines we discussed - using your palm for protein, cupped hand for carbohydrates, and thumb for fats - provide a practical starting point for portion control without the need for complicated measurements.

As you begin applying these concepts to your nutrition journey, start with the basics. Focus on including a source of protein, carbohydrates, and healthy fats at each main meal. Pay attention to how different combinations make you feel. Are you staying energized throughout the day? Do you feel satisfied after meals? These observations will help you fine-tune your macro balance to support your individual needs and goals.

In the chapters ahead, we'll build upon this foundation, exploring how to calculate your specific macro needs, create practical meal plans, and adapt your approach for different activities and goals. For now, focus on understanding these basic building blocks and practicing the simple portion control methods we've discussed.

Your journey to macro mastery has begun with understanding these fundamental nutrients. Like learning any new skill, mastering macro-nutrition takes practice and patience. Start with the basics we've covered here, and remember that small, consistent changes in how you balance these nutrients can lead to significant improvements in your energy, health, and overall well-being.

As we move forward, keep in mind that there's no one-size-fits-all approach to nutrition. The principles we've explored in this chapter provide a framework that you can adapt to your unique needs, preferences, and lifestyle. Whether your goal is weight management, improved athletic performance, or simply better overall health, understanding these macronutrient basics will serve as a solid foundation for success.

Chapter 2

The Science of Calorie Counting: Making Numbers Work for You

Every time you sit down for a meal, you're not just eating food - you're fueling your body with complex biological building blocks that determine how you feel, perform, and function. Understanding these building blocks, known as macronutrients, is like learning the alphabet before writing a story - it's the fundamental knowledge that empowers you to make informed decisions about your nutrition. These fundamental elements of nutrition work in harmony within your body, each playing vital roles in everything from energy production to muscle repair and hormone regulation. By developing a clear understanding of how macronutrients function, you can make informed decisions about your food choices that support your health and fitness goals.

Think of macronutrients as the primary colors of nutrition - just as an artist combines red, blue, and yellow to create countless hues, your body combines proteins, carbohydrates, and fats to perform numerous essential functions. When balanced correctly, these nutrients make a symphony of biological processes that keep you energized, focused, and performing at your best.

During my early days as a nutrition enthusiast, I found myself standing in my kitchen, overwhelmed by the conflicting information I'd read about macronutrients. I had a counter full of various foods - chicken breast, sweet potatoes, avocados, and brown rice - but I felt paralyzed about how to combine them effectively. One evening, while preparing dinner for my family, I decided to approach it differently. Instead of seeing these ingredients as just food, I began thinking of them as pieces of a puzzle. The chicken breast became my protein building blocks for muscle repair, the sweet potatoes transformed into energy-giving carbohydrates, and the avocados represented essential fats for hormone balance and nutrient absorption. This simple shift in perspective not only made meal planning more intuitive but also helped me explain these concepts to my clients. Now, when I teach others about macronutrients, I use this same approach - breaking down complex nutrition science into tangible, real-world examples that anyone can understand and apply to their daily lives.

As we delve deeper into each macronutrient, you'll discover how they individually contribute to your body's functions and how they work together to create optimal health. Whether your goal is weight management, athletic performance, or simply better overall health, understanding these nutritional building blocks is your first step toward achieving sustainable results.

This chapter will equip you with practical knowledge about the role of proteins in muscle maintenance and repair, the function of carbohydrates as your body's preferred energy source, and the importance of fats in hormone production and nutrient absorption. You'll learn how to identify good sources of each macronutrient and understand how to balance them effectively in your daily meals.

Understanding Your Basic Metabolic Rate (BMR) and Daily Energy Needs

Your body is like a car that's always running - even when you're completely still, it's burning fuel to keep your heart beating, your lungs breathing, and your cells functioning. This constant energy expenditure is known as your Basic Metabolic Rate (BMR), and understanding it is crucial to mastering your nutrition needs.

Think of your BMR as your body's baseline energy requirement—the number of calories you'd burn if you stayed in bed all day. It accounts for about 60-70% of your daily calorie needs and is influenced by several factors, including your age, gender, height, weight, and body composition. The more muscle mass you have, the higher your BMR tends to be, as muscle tissue requires more energy to maintain than fat tissue.

When I first started learning about BMR, I was working with a client named Sarah who couldn't understand why her friend could eat significantly more than her while maintaining the same weight. After calculating their respective BMRs, the answer became clear - Sarah's friend, who had more muscle mass and was several inches taller, had a BMR nearly 400 calories higher than Sarah's. This revelation helped Sarah understand why copying her friend's eating habits wasn't working for her goals.

To calculate your BMR, several formulas are available; however, one of the most widely used is the Harris-Benedict equation. Although the exact formula may seem complex, numerous online calculators can help you quickly determine your BMR. However, remember that this is just a starting point - your actual energy needs will vary based on your activity level.

Your total daily energy expenditure (TDEE) is based on your basal metabolic rate (BMR) and factors in your activity level. This includes both structured exercise and non-exercise activity thermogenesis (NEAT) - all the movement you do throughout the day that isn't formal exercise, like walking to your car, doing household chores, or fidgeting at your desk.

- Sedentary (little or no exercise): BMR x 1.2

- Lightly active (light exercise 1-3 days/week): BMR x 1.375

- Moderately active (moderate exercise 3-5 days/week): BMR x 1.55

- Very active (challenging exercise 6-7 days/week): BMR x 1.725

- Extra active (challenging exercise and physical job): BMR x 1.9

Understanding your BMR and TDEE provides the foundation for setting realistic nutrition goals. If you're aiming to maintain your weight, you'll want to consume approximately the same number of calories as your Total Daily Energy Expenditure (TDEE). For weight loss, you might create a moderate deficit, while muscle gain typically requires a small surplus.

However, these calculations aren't set in stone. Your body is dynamic, and your energy needs can fluctuate based on various factors, including stress levels, sleep quality, hormonal fluctuations, and even the temperature outside. That's why it's essential to view these numbers as starting points rather than absolute rules.

I encourage my clients to track their energy intake and weight trends over several weeks, making adjustments based on their progress and how they feel. Remember, the goal isn't to hit exact numbers every day, but rather to understand your body's general energy needs and respond accordingly.

Keeping track of your BMR and daily energy needs doesn't mean you need to become a human calculator. Start by establishing a baseline understanding of your needs, then learn to adjust intuitively based on your activity level and goals. This knowledge becomes particularly valuable when we begin discussing macro ratios and meal planning in later chapters.

The Energy Balance Equation: Calories In vs. Calories Out

At its core, weight management follows a fundamental principle known as the energy balance equation - calories in versus calories out. This concept, while simple in theory, is often misunderstood in practice. Think of your body's energy balance like a bank account - deposits are the calories you consume through food and drinks. At the same time, withdrawals are the calories your body burns through essential functions and physical activity.

When I first started teaching nutrition workshops, I used a simple demonstration that resonated with many participants. I would bring two clear jars—one representing daily calorie intake and another representing calorie expenditure. As we added marbles representing calories consumed and removed ones for calories burned, the visual helped people understand how slight daily differences in energy balance could accumulate over time.

Your body is constantly using energy, even when you're completely still. This baseline energy expenditure, combined with your daily activities, creates your total daily energy needs. When you consume the same number of calories as you burn, you maintain your weight. Consume more than you burn, and your body stores the excess energy, typically as fat tissue. Burn more than you consume, and your body taps into stored energy reserves for fuel.

However, the energy balance equation isn't as simple as basic mathematics. Your body is a complex biological system that adapts to changes in energy intake and expenditure. When you reduce your calorie intake, your body may respond by becoming more efficient with its energy use, which can result in a slight decrease in your metabolic rate. Similarly, increasing physical activity often leads to improved metabolic efficiency over time.

Consider these key components of the energy balance equation:

- Calories In: Food and beverage consumption

- Calories Out: Basic metabolic rate (BMR)

- Physical activity (both exercise and daily movement)

- Thermic effect of food (energy used for digestion)

- Non-exercise activity thermogenesis (NEAT)

Understanding this equation helps explain why small, consistent changes often lead to better long-term results than dramatic short-term adjustments. For instance, creating a modest daily deficit of 500 calories through a combination of reduced intake and increased physical activity is generally more sustainable than severely restricting calories or engaging in excessive exercise.

I once worked with a client named Marco who was frustrated by his lack of progress despite what he thought was a significant calorie deficit. Through careful tracking, we discovered that while he diligently counted calories Monday through Friday, his weekend habits created a surplus that offset his weekday deficit. By understanding the energy balance equation, we were able to make adjustments that created a consistent, moderate deficit throughout the week.

The energy balance equation also explains why different approaches to weight management can be successful as long as they create the appropriate energy balance. Whether someone follows a low-carb, plant-based, or Mediterranean-style diet, weight changes ultimately depend on the balance between energy intake and expenditure.

However, it's crucial to remember that while calories matter, they're not the only consideration in a healthy nutrition plan. The quality of those calories has a significant impact on your health, energy levels, and ability to maintain a consistent energy balance. Nutrient-dense foods typically provide better satiety, helping you naturally maintain appropriate portion sizes.

When applying the energy balance equation to your nutrition plan, start by establishing a baseline understanding of your current intake and expenditure. This doesn't require precise calorie counting - even rough estimates can help you identify patterns and make informed adjustments. Focus on creating sustainable habits that support your desired energy balance rather than pursuing perfect mathematical precision.

Remember that your energy needs aren't static - they change based on factors like activity level, stress, sleep quality, and even the weather. The key is learning to adjust your intake based on these variables while maintaining an overall balance that supports your goals. This flexible approach allows you to navigate real-world situations while staying aligned with your long-term nutrition objectives.

Digital Tools and Apps: Choosing the Right Tracking Method

In today's digital age, tracking your nutrition has never been more accessible, with countless apps and tools available at your fingertips. However, finding the proper tracking method isn't about choosing the most sophisticated app - it's about selecting a tool that fits seamlessly into your lifestyle and supports your nutrition goals.

When I first started teaching macro tracking, I worked with a client named Sally who had downloaded five different nutrition apps but felt overwhelmed by their complexity. Together, we evaluated her needs and discovered that a simple note-taking app combined with a basic food database worked better for her lifestyle than the more complex tracking options she'd been struggling with.

When choosing a digital tracking tool, consider these essential features:

- User-friendly food database with accurate macro information

- Quick entry options for frequently consumed meals

- Ability to create and save custom recipes

- Barcode scanning capability for packaged foods

- Progress tracking and reporting features

- Meal planning functionality

- Integration with other health apps or devices

The key is finding a balance between functionality and simplicity. The most effective tracking tool is one that you use consistently. Some people thrive with comprehensive apps that track every detail, while others prefer more straightforward options that focus on basic macro tracking.

One approach I often recommend to beginners is to start with a basic food logging app and gradually explore more advanced features as they become comfortable with tracking. This prevents the common pitfall of becoming overwhelmed by too many features too soon.

Remember that digital tools should support your nutrition journey, not control it. While apps can provide valuable insights and make tracking more convenient, they shouldn't become a source of stress or obsession. I encourage my clients to use technology as a learning tool, gradually developing an intuitive understanding of portion sizes and macro content in everyday foods.

Many of my successful clients combine digital tracking with practical strategies, such as using hand portions for quick estimates when eating out or taking photos of meals for later logging. This hybrid approach allows for flexibility while maintaining awareness of macro intake.

When setting up your chosen tracking tool, take time to customize it to your needs. Most apps allow you to set personalized macro goals, create meal templates, and save favorite foods. This initial setup investment can save hours in the long run and make daily tracking much more manageable.

I've found that the most successful long-term trackers often use their digital tools as a reference point rather than a strict rulebook. They might track meticulously during the week but estimate on weekends, or use detailed tracking when trying new foods but rely on saved meals and quick entries for familiar options.

Whichever tool you choose, remember that consistency matters more than perfection. A simple app used regularly will provide better insights than a sophisticated tool used sporadically. Start with the basics, focus on developing sustainable habits, and let your tracking method evolve with your nutrition journey.

As you become more comfortable with tracking, you may naturally gravitate toward certain features or wish for additional functionality. Don't be afraid to switch tools or combine different methods to create a system that works best for you. The goal is to make tracking a helpful part of your nutrition strategy, not an additional source of stress in your daily routine.

Common Calorie Counting Pitfalls and How to Avoid Them

While calorie counting can be an effective tool for managing nutrition and achieving health goals, several common pitfalls can derail progress or lead to frustration. Understanding these challenges and having strategies to overcome them is crucial for long-term success.

One of the most frequent mistakes I see in my nutrition practice is underestimating portion sizes. I recall working with a client, Lisa, who meticulously tracked her food intake but wasn't seeing the expected results. When we reviewed her food diary together, we discovered that she was significantly underestimating her portions, particularly with calorie-dense foods such as nuts, oils, and spreads. To address this, we began using essential kitchen tools and visual references - a tablespoon of peanut butter should resemble a poker chip, while a serving of nuts should fit in a small, cupped palm.

Another common pitfall is the "health halo" effect, which assumes that healthy foods are automatically low in calories. Foods like avocados, nuts, olive oil, and granola are nutrient-rich but also calorie-dense. During one of my workshops, a participant was surprised to learn that her daily smoothie bowl, topped with granola, coconut, and nut butter, contained more calories than the breakfast she was trying to replace.

- Forgetting to track beverages and cooking oils

- Not accounting for condiments and sauces

- Eyeballing portions instead of measuring

- Neglecting to track small bites and tastes

- Assuming restaurant portions match standard serving sizes

Accurate tracking requires attention to these often-overlooked sources of calories. I encourage my clients to keep a food scale and measuring tools handy, especially when first learning portion sizes. Over time, this practice develops a better sense of portion control without needing to measure everything.

The weekend effect is another significant pitfall: maintaining careful tracking during the week but letting it slip on weekends. This pattern can easily undo progress made during the week. Instead of abandoning tracking entirely on weekends, I recommend a flexible approach that maintains awareness while allowing for social events and special occasions.

Many people also fall into the trap of not adjusting their calorie goals as their body composition changes. As you lose weight, your caloric needs typically decrease, requiring periodic adjustments to maintain progress. Regular reassessment of your calorie targets, usually every 10-15 pounds of weight change, helps prevent plateaus.

One particularly destructive pitfall is the all-or-nothing mindset. I worked with a client named Tom who would abandon his tracking thoroughly after one unplanned meal or snack, leading to days of unmonitored eating. We worked on developing a more balanced approach, understanding that one off-track meal doesn't negate overall progress.

To avoid these common pitfalls, consider these practical strategies:

- Use measuring tools consistently until you develop reliable portion awareness

- Track everything immediately rather than trying to remember at day's end

- Keep a digital food scale at home and work, if possible

- Take photos of meals for later reference

- Pre-log meals when planning your day

Remember that successful calorie counting isn't about perfection - it's about consistency and awareness. Start by focusing on the most significant sources of calories in your diet, then gradually increase accuracy as you become more comfortable with tracking. This approach helps prevent the overwhelm that often leads to abandoning tracking altogether.

Another crucial aspect is learning to navigate social situations while maintaining awareness of calorie intake. Rather than declining social invitations or stressing about exact measurements, develop strategies for estimating portions and making informed choices. This might mean checking restaurant menus in advance, eating a small protein-rich snack before events, or simply focusing on mindful eating when exact tracking isn't practical.

Lastly, avoid the pitfall of using calorie counting as a punishment rather than a tool for awareness and self-improvement. The goal is to develop a healthy relationship with food while working toward your health objectives. If you find yourself becoming overly preoccupied with tracking or feeling guilty about your food choices, it's essential to step back and reassess your approach. Sometimes, taking a brief break from detailed tracking and focusing on mindful eating can help reset your perspective while maintaining awareness of portion sizes and food choices.

Flexible Tracking: Making Calorie Counting Sustainable

Sustainable calorie tracking isn't about perfect precision - it's about finding a balanced approach that you can maintain long-term while living a whole and enjoyable life. Through my years of nutrition coaching, I've discovered that the most successful individuals are those who adopt flexible tracking methods that bend with life's challenges without breaking.

I often share the story of my client Amy, who initially approached calorie tracking with an all-or-nothing mindset. She would meticulously weigh every morsel of food at home but abandon tracking entirely when eating out or traveling for work. Together, we developed a more sustainable approach using what I call the "80/20 method" - tracking with precision when possible, while using practical estimation techniques for the remaining situations.

The key to flexible tracking lies in developing a toolkit of strategies that you can adapt to different situations:

- Use kitchen scales and measuring tools at home to build portion awareness

- Learn hand-portion estimations for when precise measuring isn't practical

- Take photos of meals for later reference and logging

- Create a database of commonly eaten meals for quick logging

- Develop rough estimates for restaurant portions based on visual cues

One of the most effective ways to maintain sustainable tracking is to establish a baseline of go-to meals and snacks that you enjoy and are familiar with, knowing their caloric content. This creates a foundation of reliable options while allowing flexibility for special occasions or unexpected situations.

I encourage my clients to think of calorie tracking as a skill that develops over time, much like learning to play a musical instrument. Initially, you might need to focus intently on every note (or in this case, every gram and calorie). Still, eventually, you develop an intuitive sense of portion sizes and caloric content that becomes second nature.

Another crucial aspect of sustainable tracking is understanding that perfection isn't necessary for progress. If you can't track a meal precisely, making an educated estimate is better than abandoning tracking altogether. I teach my clients to use benchmark meals—well-tracked meals they eat regularly—as reference points for estimating similar meals in different situations.

The concept of "calorie bracketing" can also be helpful for sustainable tracking. This involves creating reasonably high and low estimates for meals when exact counting isn't possible. For example, if you're eating at a restaurant where nutritional information isn't available, you might estimate that your grilled chicken salad contains between 400 and 600 calories. This range acknowledges the uncertainty while keeping you mindful of portion sizes.

Flexible tracking also means adapting your approach based on your current circumstances. During periods of routine, such as typical workweeks, you may track more precisely. During holidays, travel, or special events, you might shift to more general guidelines and estimations while maintaining awareness of portion sizes and food choices.

Remember that the goal of tracking isn't to create a perfect log of every calorie consumed - it's to develop awareness of your eating patterns and make informed choices that support your health goals. Some days, you'll track everything precisely; others, you'll estimate; and occasionally, you might not track at all. What matters is maintaining a consistent approach over time while allowing for the natural ebb and flow of life.

I've found that clients who embrace flexible tracking tend to maintain their habits longer and achieve better long-term results than those who insist on perfect precision. They learn to trust their judgment, make educated estimates when necessary, and most importantly, maintain a healthy relationship with food while working toward their goals.

To make your tracking more sustainable, start by identifying the situations where precise monitoring is most challenging for you. Then, develop specific strategies for those scenarios. For instance, if you frequently eat at restaurants, you might create a quick reference guide of typical meals at your favorite places. If you travel often, you may establish a set of essential foods and meal choices that you can rely on while away from home.

The key is to strike a balance between accuracy and practicality that suits your lifestyle. With practice, you'll develop the confidence to make informed estimates when needed while maintaining enough precision to support your nutrition goals. Remember, sustainable tracking is about progress, not perfection, and the best tracking system is one you can maintain consistently over time. As we conclude this foundational chapter on macronutrients, let's reflect on the essential building blocks that form the basis of our nutrition. Just as we began with my kitchen revelation about seeing ingredients as puzzle pieces rather than just food, I hope you're now viewing your meals through a new lens—one that recognizes the vital roles of proteins, carbohydrates, and fats in supporting your body's functions.

Through our exploration of Basic Metabolic Rate (BMR) and daily energy needs, we've discovered that understanding your body's unique energy requirements isn't about memorizing complex formulas, but rather about recognizing how your lifestyle, activity level, and individual characteristics influence your nutritional needs. The energy balance equation we discussed demonstrates that while calories matter, they're just one part of a larger picture that includes the quality and composition of those calories.

Remember our discussion about digital tracking tools and common pitfalls? These insights weren't just theoretical—they came from actual experiences of learning to navigate nutrition tracking in practical, sustainable ways. Whether you choose to use sophisticated apps or simple hand measurements, the goal is to find methods that work for your lifestyle while maintaining awareness of your macro intake.

As we move forward in your macro-nutrition journey, keep in mind that this knowledge forms the foundation for all the practical applications we'll explore in later chapters. Understanding these basics—how proteins support muscle maintenance, how carbohydrates fuel your daily activities, and how fats enable vital bodily functions—will help you make informed decisions about your nutrition.

You're now equipped with the fundamental knowledge needed to begin personalizing your macro approach. Remember, just as my experience of breaking down that family dinner into its macro components led to better understanding, your journey of implementing these principles will lead to your insights and discoveries.

In the following chapters, we'll build upon this foundation, exploring how to apply these concepts to meal planning, adjusting your macro intake for different goals, and navigating real-world challenges while maintaining your nutrition targets. But for now, take pride in knowing you've mastered the fundamental building blocks of nutrition - knowledge that will serve as your compass throughout your wellness journey.

Chapter 3

Mastering Macro Balance: Your Personalized Nutrition Formula

Numbers tell stories, and in nutrition, calories tell the story of energy - how much we consume and how much we use. While many people view calorie counting as a dreaded math exercise, I'm going to show you how understanding these numbers can become an intuitive part of your wellness journey, much like checking your bank account helps you manage your finances. Understanding these numbers and how they work together can revolutionize your approach to nutrition, making it more intuitive and less intimidating. Think of calorie counting as learning a new language - at first, the numbers may seem foreign and complex. Still, with practice, they become second nature, allowing you to make informed choices effortlessly.

In my years of nutrition coaching, I've seen how proper calorie awareness can transform lives when approached with the right mindset. During a nutrition workshop I was hosting, a participant named Sarah approached me with tears in her eyes. She had been meticulously counting calories for months, weighing every morsel of food and logging it into her tracking app, but the process had become all-consuming. Her social life was suffering because she avoided restaurants where she couldn't precisely calculate calories, and family meals had become a source of anxiety. Together, we developed a more balanced approach. I showed her how to estimate portions using hand measurements and how to make educated guesses when eating out. We focused on understanding general portion sizes and calorie ranges rather than exact numbers.

Within weeks, Sarah reported feeling liberated. She was still aware of her calorie intake, but no longer let it control her life. Her story perfectly illustrates why I advocate for an approach to calorie counting that emphasizes awareness over perfectionism. Six months later, she not only maintained her health goals but also rediscovered the joy of sharing meals with friends and family, proving that effective calorie counting doesn't require sacrificing one's quality of life.

In this chapter, we'll explore how to make calorie counting work for you, not against you. We'll discover practical tools and techniques that simplify the process, making it an empowering part of your nutrition journey rather than a source of stress. You'll learn how to calculate your personal caloric needs, understand the relationship between calories and energy balance, and develop sustainable tracking habits that fit your lifestyle.

Most importantly, we'll focus on building a healthy relationship with numbers while maintaining the joy of eating. Whether you're new to calorie counting or seeking to adopt a more balanced approach, this chapter will equip you with the knowledge and strategies to make informed decisions about your nutrition without becoming overly focused on the numbers.

Calculating Your Macro Ratios: Beyond Basic Formulas

When it comes to calculating your macro ratios, there's more to consider than just plugging numbers into a basic formula. While standard calculations provide a starting point, your optimal macro balance depends on various factors unique to you, including your body composition, activity level, lifestyle, and specific goals, all of which play crucial roles in determining your ideal macro distribution.

Let's start with the fundamental principle of macro balance. While the standard recommendation often suggests a ratio of 45-65% carbohydrates, 20-35% fats, and 10-35% protein, these ranges are intentionally wide because they need to accommodate different body types and goals. Think of these ranges as a framework rather than strict rules - they're your starting point for personalization.

To illustrate this concept, let me share a story about my client Michael, an office worker who also enjoys weekend hiking. When he first started tracking macros, he followed a standard 50/30/20 split (carbs/protein/fat), but found himself lacking energy during his weekend adventures. By adjusting his carbohydrate intake higher on hiking days and maintaining a more moderate level during workdays, we created a flexible system that supported both his active and sedentary periods.

To begin calculating your personal ratios, start by determining your total daily calorie needs. Then, consider these key factors that influence your macro distribution:

- **Activity Type and Level:** Endurance activities typically require higher carbohydrate ratios, while strength training may need increased protein

- **Body Composition Goals:** Fat loss often benefits from higher protein ratios, while muscle gain might need balanced increases in both protein and carbohydrates

- **Current Body Composition:** Your existing lean mass and body fat percentage influence your macro needs

- **Daily Schedule:** Consider when you exercise and how your energy needs fluctuate throughout the day

- **Food Preferences:** Your macro ratios should accommodate foods you enjoy and can consistently include in your diet

Once you've considered these factors, you can begin fine-tuning your ratios. A practical approach is to start with these baseline calculations:

- Calculate protein needs first (typically 0.8-1.2g per pound of target body weight)

- Allocate fat intake (usually 0.3-0.5g per pound of body weight)

- Fill the remaining calories with carbohydrates

This method provides structure while allowing for personalization. Remember, these numbers are starting points, not final destinations. The key is to monitor how your body responds and make adjustments accordingly.

One effective strategy I've developed with clients is the "two-week test and adjust" method. Start with your calculated ratios and maintain them consistently for two weeks while tracking your energy levels, hunger, performance, and progress toward your goals. Make notes about how you feel during various activities and at different times of day. After two weeks, analyze this data to make informed adjustments.

For example, if you notice your energy dipping during afternoon workouts, you might need to increase your pre-workout carbohydrates. If you're consistently hungry between meals, you may need to adjust your protein or fat intake to achieve better satiety.

Remember that your macro needs aren't static - they evolve with your lifestyle and goals. During periods of intense training, you might need to increase overall intake while maintaining similar ratios. During periods of reduced activity, you may reduce your total calorie intake while maintaining a higher protein intake to help preserve muscle mass.

The most successful approach to macro calculation is one that views it as an ongoing process of refinement rather than a one-time calculation. Think of it as tuning an instrument - you start with standard tuning, but make minor adjustments based on the specific piece you're playing and the environmental conditions.

As you become more attuned to your body's responses, you'll develop an intuitive understanding of when and how to adjust your macros. This dynamic approach ensures that your nutrition plan remains effective as it adapts to your changing needs and goals.

Goal-Specific Macro Adjustments: Weight Loss, Muscle Gain, and Maintenance

Understanding how to adjust your macronutrient ratios for specific goals is like having a roadmap for your nutrition journey. Whether you're looking to lose weight, build muscle, or maintain your current composition, your macro distribution plays a crucial role in achieving these outcomes. Let's explore how to optimize your macros for each goal while maintaining a sustainable and enjoyable approach to eating.

For weight loss, the focus shifts toward creating a moderate caloric deficit while maintaining adequate protein to preserve muscle mass. A typical starting point is to increase protein to 30-35% of total calories, moderate carbohydrates to 35-40%, and keep fats at 25-30%. This distribution helps manage hunger, preserve lean tissue, and provide enough energy for daily activities. I recently worked with a client, Lisa, who struggled with previous low-calorie diets that left her feeling depleted. By adjusting her macros to emphasize protein and including strategic carbohydrate timing around her workouts, she maintained her energy levels while steadily progressing toward her weight loss goals.

Muscle gain requires a different approach, typically involving a slight caloric surplus, along with increased protein and carbohydrates, to support muscle growth and recovery. A typical starting ratio might be 25-30% protein, 45-55% carbohydrates, and 20-25% fats. The higher carbohydrate intake helps fuel intense training sessions and promotes recovery, while adequate protein provides the building blocks for new muscle tissue.

For maintenance, the goal is to find a balanced macro distribution that sustains your current body composition while supporting your activity level and lifestyle. This often means adjusting ratios based on your daily routine and energy needs. A balanced approach might start with 25-30% protein, 40-45% carbohydrates, and 25-30% fats, with adjustments made based on how your body responds.

Regardless of your goal, remember that these ratios are starting points, not rigid rules. Your optimal distribution may vary based on factors like:

- Activity level and type of exercise

- Individual metabolism and body composition

- Food preferences and dietary restrictions

- Daily schedule and lifestyle demands

- Stress levels and sleep quality

The key to successful macro adjustment is monitoring your progress and making incremental changes. Start with a baseline distribution and track your results for 2-3 weeks, noting energy levels, hunger, performance, and progress toward your goals. Make small adjustments (3-5% shifts in ratios) based on your observations.

One of my most successful clients, Tom, taught me the importance of flexible macro adjustment. As a busy professional training for his first marathon, he needed different macro ratios for training days versus rest days. We developed a dual-approach system: higher carbohydrates (50-55%) on training days to fuel his runs, and a more moderate carbohydrate intake (40-45%) on rest days, while maintaining consistent protein levels throughout the week.

When adjusting your macros for any goal, consider implementing these practical strategies:

- Plan protein intake first, as it remains essential across all goals

- Adjust carbohydrates based on activity level and timing

- Keep fats moderate but sufficient for hormone function

- Include a variety of food sources to ensure micronutrient intake

- Allow for flexibility during social occasions and special events

Remember that successful macro adjustment isn't about perfect adherence to specific numbers, but rather about creating a sustainable approach that supports your goals while fitting into your lifestyle. Monitor your progress, listen to your body's signals, and make adjustments as needed. The most effective macro distribution is one you can maintain consistently while enjoying your food choices and making progress toward your goals.

As you experiment with different macro ratios, keep a journal to note not only your numbers but also how you feel. This feedback will be invaluable in refining your approach and developing a personalized nutrition strategy that supports your specific goals while fostering a healthy relationship with food.

Activity Level and Lifestyle Considerations in Macro Planning

Your activity level and lifestyle play pivotal roles in determining your macro needs, much like how a car's fuel requirements vary depending on whether it's cruising highways or climbing mountains. Understanding how to adjust your macros based on these factors is crucial for optimizing your nutrition plan and achieving your health goals.

I learned this lesson firsthand while working with Sarah, a nurse who switched from day shifts to night shifts. Her previous macro plan, which worked flawlessly during regular hours, left her feeling sluggish and hungry during overnight work. Together, we discovered that her new schedule required different macro timing and distribution to maintain her energy levels throughout her shifts.

Your activity level significantly impacts your macro requirements in several ways:

- **Energy Needs:** Higher activity levels require increased overall calorie intake

- **Carbohydrate Requirements:** More intense activity typically demands higher carbohydrate intake

- **Protein Timing:** Active individuals often benefit from strategic protein distribution

- **Recovery Needs:** More strenuous activity requires adjusted macro ratios for optimal recovery

- **Meal Timing:** Activity schedules influence when and how you should consume different macros

To effectively plan your macros around your activity level, start by categorizing your typical daily activity. Are you:

- Sedentary (minimal exercise)

- Lightly Active (1-3 days of exercise per week)

- Moderately Active (3-5 days of exercise per week)

- Very Active (6-7 days of exercise per week)

- Extremely Active (intense exercise or physical job)

Beyond just exercise, consider your overall lifestyle factors that influence macro needs:

- **Work Schedule:** Different shifts may require adjusted meal timing

- **Stress Levels:** Higher stress might necessitate different macro distributions

- **Sleep Patterns:** Poor sleep can affect how your body processes different macronutrients

- **Travel Frequency:** Regular travel requires flexible macro planning

- **Family Commitments:** A Busy family life needs practical macro solutions

One of my clients, Mark, worked as a construction worker while also training for recreational sports leagues. His high physical demands required a unique approach to macro planning. We developed a system where he consumed higher carbohydrates during work hours for sustained energy, followed by increased protein intake in the evening to support recovery. This personalized approach considered both his job demands and training goals.

When adjusting your macros for activity level, consider these practical strategies:

- Time your carbohydrate intake around your most active periods

- Distribute protein intake evenly throughout the day

- Adjust fat intake based on energy needs and meal timing

- Plan for pre- and post-workout nutrition

- Create flexible meal options for busy days

Remember that your macro needs may vary from day to day, depending on your activity. For instance, a rest day might require fewer carbohydrates compared to a heavy training day. This dynamic approach allows your nutrition to support your changing energy demands while maintaining progress toward your goals.

Lifestyle considerations also extend to meal preparation and timing. If you're frequently on the go, you'll need strategies for portable, macro-friendly meals. If you work long hours, batch cooking and meal prep become essential tools for maintaining your macro targets.

Consider creating different macro templates for:

- Training days vs. rest days

- Work days vs. off days

- High-stress periods vs. routine

- Travel days vs. home routine

- Seasonal activity changes

The key to successful macro planning is building flexibility into your system while maintaining consistency with your overall targets. This may involve planning higher-carbohydrate meals around workouts, protein-rich snacks for busy periods, and strategic meal timing based on your daily schedule.

Remember that your activity level and lifestyle aren't static - they change with seasons, work demands, and life events. Regular reassessment of your macro needs ensures your nutrition plan continues to support your changing lifestyle while maintaining progress toward your health and fitness goals.

Fine-Tuning Your Macro Balance: Signs and Adjustments

Fine-tuning your macro balance is like adjusting the dials on a radio - small changes can make a significant difference in the quality of your results. Understanding the signs your body gives you and knowing how to make appropriate adjustments is crucial for optimizing your nutrition plan. Let's explore how to recognize these signals and make informed modifications to your macro intake.

Your body provides various indicators that your current macro balance might need adjustment. These signs can include:

- **Energy Fluctuations:** Unusual fatigue or energy crashes during the day

- **Hunger Patterns:** Feeling unusually hungry between meals or a lack of satiety

- **Exercise Performance:** Decreased strength or endurance during workouts

- **Recovery Quality:** Longer recovery times or increased muscle soreness

- **Sleep Changes:** Disrupted sleep patterns or difficulty falling asleep

- **Mood Variations:** Increased irritability or mood swings

I recently worked with a client, Jennifer, who came to me feeling constantly tired despite getting adequate sleep. After reviewing her macro intake, we discovered her carbohydrate levels were too low for her active lifestyle, leading to energy crashes in the afternoon. By gradually increasing her carbohydrate intake around her workout times while maintaining her protein levels, her energy stabilized and her performance improved.

When making macro adjustments, it's essential to follow a systematic approach. Start with small changes (5-10% shifts in ratios) and monitor their effects for at least two weeks before making additional modifications. This methodical approach helps identify which changes are truly effective for your body.

Here's a practical framework for making macro adjustments:

- **Document Current State:** Track your energy, hunger, and performance

- **Make One Change:** Adjust a single macro ratio at a time

- **Monitor Results:** Keep detailed notes on how you feel

- **Evaluate Impact:** Assess whether the change improved your symptoms

- **Fine-tune Further:** Make additional minor adjustments as needed

The timing of your macro intake can be just as important as the ratios themselves. For instance, if you're experiencing mid-workout fatigue, you might need to adjust your pre-workout carbohydrate timing rather than your overall daily carbohydrate intake.

One of the most valuable lessons I've learned in my practice is that macro adjustments often need to be seasonal. Your body's needs can change in response to the weather, stress levels, and activity patterns. During the winter months, you may need a slightly higher carbohydrate intake to maintain energy and warmth, while in summer, different adjustments may be required.

Common adjustment scenarios and solutions include:

- **Persistent Hunger:** Consider increasing protein or fiber-rich carbohydrates

- **Low Energy:** Evaluate carbohydrate timing and overall intake

- **Poor Recovery:** Review protein distribution throughout the day

- **Plateau in Progress:** Reassess overall calorie intake and macro ratios

- **Digestive Issues:** Consider the types of foods within each macro category

Remember that successful macro adjustment isn't just about the numbers - it's about creating a sustainable approach that supports your goals while maintaining a healthy relationship with food. Pay attention to how different foods within each macro category affect you. Sometimes, the source of your macros matters as much as the quantity.

When making adjustments, keep these principles in mind:

- Patience is key - give your body time to adapt to changes

- Keep detailed records of adjustments and their effects

- Consider external factors that might influence your results

- Maintain consistency with other lifestyle factors during adjustment periods

- Stay flexible and willing to make further modifications as needed

The art of fine-tuning your macro balance lies in finding the sweet spot between structure and flexibility. While it's essential to have guidelines and targets, remember that your body's needs are dynamic and can change in response to various factors. The goal is to develop an intuitive understanding of your body's signals while maintaining a structured approach to adjustments.

Through consistent monitoring and thoughtful adjustments, you'll develop a deeper understanding of how your body responds to different macro balances. This knowledge becomes invaluable as you continue your nutrition journey, enabling you to make informed decisions about your macronutrient intake that support your evolving needs and goals.

Creating Flexible Meal Templates Around Your Macro Goals

Creating flexible meal templates is like building a customizable wardrobe - you need versatile pieces that can be mixed and matched to suit different occasions while maintaining your style. In the context of macro nutrition, these templates serve as your foundation for consistent, sustainable eating that meets your nutritional goals while adapting to your daily life.

When I first started developing meal templates with my clients, I worked with a busy mother named Rachel who struggled to maintain her macro goals while cooking for her family. Together, we created a system of interchangeable meal components that could be adjusted to suit both her macro needs and her family's preferences. This approach transformed her meal planning from a daily struggle into an effortless routine.

To begin creating your flexible meal templates, start with these fundamental building blocks:

- Protein Sources: Lean meats, fish, eggs, legumes, dairy

- Carbohydrate Options: Whole grains, starchy vegetables, fruits

- Healthy Fats: Nuts, seeds, oils, avocados

- Volume Foods: Non-starchy vegetables, leafy greens

The key to successful template creation lies in understanding portion sizes and their corresponding macro contributions. Rather than measuring everything precisely, use these practical portion guidelines:

- Protein: Palm-sized portions (roughly 20-30g protein)

- Carbohydrates: Cupped hand portions (roughly 20-30g carbs)

- Fats: Thumb-sized portions (roughly 7-9g fat)

- Vegetables: Fist-sized portions

With these building blocks and portion guidelines in mind, you can create various meal templates that fit different scenarios. For example, a basic template might include:

Breakfast Template:

- 1-2 protein portions

- 1 carbohydrate portion

- 1 fat portion

- 1 vegetable portion

This template could translate into multiple meal variations:

- Eggs with oatmeal, nuts, and spinach

- Greek yogurt with fruit, seeds, and berries

- Protein smoothie with banana, nut butter, and greens

The beauty of template-based meal planning lies in its flexibility. During my years of nutrition coaching, I've found that clients who use templates rather than rigid meal plans are more likely to maintain their macro goals in the long term. They learn to adapt their meals to different situations while keeping their nutrition on track.

One particularly effective strategy is creating themed templates for different days or situations:

- Quick Breakfast Templates (15 minutes or less)

- Meal Prep Templates (batch cooking friendly)

- On-the-Go Templates (portable options)

- Family Dinner Templates (crowd-pleasing choices)

- Post-Workout Templates (recovery-focused)

Remember that your templates should reflect your personal preferences and lifestyle needs. A template that works perfectly for someone else might need adjustment to fit your schedule, cooking abilities, or food preferences.

To make your templates truly flexible, include swap options within each category. For example, if your template calls for a palm-sized portion of protein, maintain a list of interchangeable options:

- Chicken breast

- Fish fillet

- Tofu block

- Legume mixture

- Greek yogurt

This approach ensures you're never left without options when certain ingredients are unavailable or don't appeal to you on a particular day.

One of my clients, Dan, used this system to maintain his macro goals while traveling for work. He created simple, hotel-room-friendly templates using portable protein sources, easily accessible carbohydrates, and minimal preparation requirements. This flexibility allowed him to maintain consistency with his nutrition goals, even when he was away from his usual routine.

As you develop your templates, consider creating seasonal variations that account for food availability and your changing preferences throughout the year. Summer templates might include more fresh, raw ingredients, while winter templates could focus on warming, cooked options.

Remember that successful template creation is an iterative process. Begin with basic templates and adjust them according to your experience and specific needs. Pay attention to which combinations keep you satisfied, energized, and enjoying your meals while meeting your macro targets.

The goal isn't to create perfect meals every time, but rather to have a reliable system that makes macro-balanced eating achievable in various situations. Your templates should serve as helpful guidelines rather than rigid rules, allowing you to maintain your nutrition goals while adapting to life's ever-changing circumstances. As we conclude this chapter on the science of calorie counting, it's important to remember that numbers are tools, not masters. Throughout this chapter, we've explored how understanding calories can empower rather than restrict, guide rather than control. From learning to calculate your personal needs to developing practical tracking strategies, you now have the foundation to make informed decisions about your nutrition.

The journey of Sarah, whom we met earlier in this chapter, reminds us that successful calorie awareness isn't about perfect precision but about finding a sustainable approach that enhances rather than diminishes our quality of life. Her transformation from obsessive tracking to confident estimation demonstrates how the right mindset and tools can make calorie management an empowering part of your wellness journey.

Remember these key takeaways as you move forward:

- Calories are information, not judgment - they help us understand our energy balance

- Flexible tracking methods can be as effective as precise measurements

- Sustainable success comes from finding a balance between awareness and enjoyment

- Your caloric needs are unique and may change with different life circumstances

- The goal is progress, not perfection

As you begin applying these concepts to your own life, start with small, manageable changes. Focus on understanding portion sizes and energy balance rather than striving for exact numbers. Trust that with practice, this knowledge will become more intuitive, allowing you to make confident choices while maintaining a healthy relationship with food.

In the next chapter, we'll build on this foundation as we explore how to personalize your macro ratios for optimal results. The understanding of calories you've gained here will be invaluable as we delve deeper into the art and science of macronutrition. Remember, every step you take toward better understanding your nutrition is progress, and even small changes can lead to significant improvements in your overall health and wellness.

Chapter 4

---^---

Smart Tracking Strategies:
Tools and Techniques for Success

Numbers tell stories, and in nutrition, calories tell the story of your body's energy balance. While many people view calorie counting as a tedious mathematical exercise, I will show you how these simple numbers can become powerful tools in your journey toward better health. These numbers, when appropriately understood, become powerful allies in achieving your health and fitness goals rather than intimidating obstacles. They tell us important stories about our energy needs, helping us make informed decisions about our nutrition without becoming slaves to mathematical precision. Just as we learn to manage our finances by understanding basic budgeting, mastering calorie awareness helps us create a sustainable approach to nutrition that supports our well-being.

Like many aspects of nutrition science, calorie counting has often been overcomplicated and misunderstood. Some view it as an all-or-nothing practice, believing they must meticulously track every morsel or abandon the concept entirely. Others see it as a punishment rather than a tool for empowerment. The reality lies somewhere in between - it's about developing awareness and understanding that serves your goals while maintaining a healthy relationship with food.

During a nutrition workshop I was hosting, a participant named Sarah approached me with tears of frustration. She had been meticulously counting every calorie for months, measuring even the smallest portions with a food scale, and logging everything in multiple apps. Her dedication to precision had turned meals into mathematical equations, stealing the joy from eating and social gatherings. Together, we worked to shift her perspective from rigid number-crunching to practical awareness. I showed her how to estimate portions using hand measurements and how to create balanced plates without needing a calculator. Six months later, Sarah sent me a photo of herself enjoying a birthday dinner with friends, beaming as she told me how liberating it felt to understand calories without being controlled by them. Her story perfectly illustrates why I'm passionate about teaching people how to make numbers work for them, rather than controlling them.

In this chapter, we'll explore how to transform calorie counting from a dreaded chore into an intuitive tool that enhances your nutrition journey. You'll learn practical methods for understanding your energy needs, simple strategies for tracking without obsession, and flexible approaches that work in real-world situations. Whether you're new to calorie awareness or seeking to cultivate a healthier relationship with tracking, you'll learn how to make these numbers work for your unique lifestyle and goals.

Remember, the goal isn't to achieve mathematical perfection in your daily intake, but rather to develop a practical understanding that guides your food choices while maintaining the joy of eating. Through this chapter, you'll learn how to utilize calorie awareness as a tool for empowerment rather than restriction, enabling you to make informed decisions about your nutrition while maintaining a balanced and enjoyable relationship with food.

Digital Tracking Tools: Choosing and Using Nutrition Apps Effectively

In today's digital age, tracking your nutrition has become more accessible than ever before. With countless apps available at our fingertips, the challenge isn't finding a tracking tool - it's choosing the right one that fits seamlessly into your lifestyle. When I first started exploring nutrition apps, I was overwhelmed by the options, and I've seen many clients face the same confusion. The key is finding a balance between functionality and usability that works for you.

When selecting a nutrition tracking app, consider these essential features:

- A comprehensive food database with accurate macro information

- The ability to save favorite meals and create custom recipes

- Quick-add options for frequently consumed foods

- User-friendly interface with minimal clicking required

- Progress tracking and reporting capabilities

- Barcode scanning functionality for packaged foods

While having these features is important, what matters most is how well the app integrates into your daily routine. I've found that the most successful tracking experiences come from apps that feel intuitive and don't require excessive time investment.

One of my clients, Marcus, struggled with nutrition tracking until we found an app that matched his tech-savvy nature and busy lifestyle. As a software developer, he appreciated apps with clean interfaces and quick input methods. We discovered that an app with a robust barcode scanner and the ability to create meal templates significantly reduced his tracking time from 30 minutes to just 5 minutes daily.

However, technology should serve as a tool, not a taskmaster. I encourage my clients to use apps as guides rather than strict rulers. The goal is to develop awareness and understanding of your nutrition, not to become dependent on digital tracking forever. Think of nutrition apps as training wheels - they provide support and guidance while you're learning, but eventually, you'll develop the intuition to make informed choices without constant digital input.

When starting with a new tracking app, follow these implementation strategies:

- Begin by tracking just one meal per day to build the habit gradually

- Use the first week to explore the app's features without worrying about hitting specific macro targets

- Create a database of your commonly eaten meals for quick future reference

- Set aside specific times for logging meals rather than tracking as you eat

- Use the app's reminder features to establish consistent tracking habits

Remember that no app is perfect, and there's often a learning curve when starting with any new tool. The key is to find an app that you'll use consistently rather than one with every possible feature but a complicated interface.

One particularly effective strategy I've developed with clients is the "batch logging" approach. Instead of logging every meal in real-time, set aside 5-10 minutes in the morning to pre-log your planned meals for the day. This not only saves time but also helps with meal planning and staying on track with your macro goals. You can constantly adjust entries later if your actual meals differ from what you planned.

As you become more comfortable with your chosen app, explore its advanced features to enhance your tracking experience. Many apps offer meal planning capabilities, grocery list generation, and trend analysis, providing valuable insights into your nutritional patterns. However, don't feel pressured to use every feature - focus on the tools that provide the most value for your specific needs and goals.

The most important aspect of digital tracking is maintaining a healthy relationship with the process. If you find yourself becoming obsessive about logging every morsel or feeling anxiety when you can't track perfectly, it's time to step back and reassess your approach. The goal is to utilize technology to support your nutritional journey, not to let it dominate your relationship with food.

Manual Tracking Methods: From Food Journals to Photo Logs

While digital tools have revolutionized nutrition tracking, there is something powerful about traditional, manual tracking methods that can enhance our awareness and connection with our food choices. In my years of coaching, I've found that some clients prefer the tangible nature of physical tracking methods, finding them more mindful and less overwhelming than their digital counterparts.

The simplest form of manual tracking starts with a basic food journal. This can be any notebook where you record your meals, portions, and timing. The act of physically writing down what you eat creates a different kind of awareness than tapping entries into an app. I've observed that the simple act of putting pen to paper often prompts people to be more thoughtful about their food choices and more aware of patterns in their eating habits.

One of my favorite manual tracking methods is the photo log, which involves simply taking pictures of your meals before eating them. This visual diary can be incredibly revealing, showing portion sizes, meal composition, and eating patterns over time. I had a client, Rebecca, who struggled with portion control until she started photographing her meals. The visual evidence helped her recognize that her dinner portions had gradually increased over time, leading to unconscious overeating.

Here are some effective manual tracking methods to consider:

- Food journals with detailed meal descriptions and timing

- Photo logs with before and after meal pictures

- Template-based tracking sheets for everyday meals

- Hand-drawn portion guides and meal planning templates

- Weekly meal planning calendars with macro breakdowns

One particularly effective manual tracking technique I've developed with clients is the 'plate mapping' method. Using a simple circle divided into quarters, you can quickly sketch out your meals, showing the proportion of proteins, carbohydrates, and vegetables. This visual approach helps develop an intuitive understanding of portion sizes and macro balance without the need for precise measurements.

The beauty of manual tracking lies in its flexibility and personalization. You can create custom templates tailored to your specific needs and goals. For instance, I worked with a client who developed a color-coding system in her food journal - green for protein sources, yellow for carbohydrates, and blue for healthy fats. This simple visual system helped her maintain macro balance without getting bogged down in exact numbers.

Manual tracking also offers unique benefits for mindful eating. The process of writing down or drawing your meals creates natural pause points, encouraging more conscious food choices. It's harder to mindlessly snack when you know you'll need to document it in your journal. This increased awareness often leads to better food choices and more intentional eating habits.

For those who enjoy creativity, bullet journal-style tracking can turn nutrition monitoring into an engaging activity. Some of my clients have created beautiful meal planning spreads that combine functionality with artistic expression. These personalized tracking systems often become cherished tools that enhance their nutrition journey rather than feeling like a chore.

However, it's important to remember that any tracking method, manual or digital, should serve as a tool for awareness rather than a source of stress. If you find yourself becoming too rigid with your documentation, it's okay to scale back or try a different approach. The goal is to develop a sustainable system that enhances your nutrition journey without dominating it.

One practical hybrid approach combines weekly manual planning with daily photo documentation. You might sketch out your meal plan for the week in a journal, then use photos to track your actual meals. This combination offers both structure and flexibility, creating a visual record of your nutritional journey.

Remember, the most effective tracking method is the one you use consistently. Whether you prefer the simplicity of an essential food journal or the creativity of a bullet journal system, choose a method that feels natural and sustainable for your lifestyle. Manual tracking can be as straightforward or as detailed as you need it to be - the key is finding what works for you and supports your nutrition goals without adding unnecessary stress to your life.

Batch Tracking and Meal Template Strategies

One of the most powerful strategies I've discovered for maintaining consistent macro tracking is the concept of batch tracking and meal templates. This approach not only saves time but also reduces the mental energy required for managing daily nutrition. Think of it as meal prep for your tracking - setting up systems in advance that make daily execution almost effortless.

When I first introduced batch tracking to my client Maria, a busy executive with three children, she was skeptical. She struggled to find time to track her meals, often forgetting to log her food until days later. Together, we developed a system where she would pre-log her common breakfast and lunch combinations as meal templates. Within weeks, her tracking consistency improved dramatically, and she reported feeling less stressed about her nutrition management.

Here are the key components of an effective batch tracking system:

- Pre-planned meal combinations with complete macro breakdowns

- Quick-access templates for common meals and snacks

- Standardized portion sizes for regular ingredients

- Weekly meal rotation schedules

- Flexible substitution options for each template

The beauty of meal templates lies in their versatility and efficiency. Instead of tracking individual ingredients every time you eat, you can quickly select pre-configured meals that you know fit your macro targets. This approach is particularly valuable for meals that tend to follow a similar pattern, such as breakfast or lunch at work.

One effective strategy I teach clients is the 'base template' approach. Start by creating templates for your most frequently consumed meals, then add variation options that maintain similar macro ratios. For example, a breakfast template might include a protein source, a complex carbohydrate, and a healthy fat. While the specific foods might change - from eggs to protein powder, and from oats to whole-grain toast - the macro balance remains consistent.

Implementing batch tracking effectively requires some initial setup time, but the long-term benefits far outweigh this investment. I recommend starting with a weekly planning session where you outline your main meals and snacks for the week ahead. During this time, you can pre-log your planned meals, create new templates as needed, and ensure your macro targets are appropriately distributed throughout the day.

Template creation follows a simple but effective structure:

- Identify your most common meals and meal combinations

- Calculate and save the macro breakdowns for these standard meals

- Create variation options that maintain similar macro ratios

- Include portion adjustments for different calorie needs

- Add notes about possible substitutions

The power of this system lies in its ability to adapt to real-life situations while maintaining a structured approach. For instance, if your lunch template includes a turkey sandwich with specific toppings, you can easily substitute the turkey with chicken or tuna while maintaining the overall macro balance. This flexibility ensures that your tracking system remains flexible rather than breaking down when faced with normal dietary variations.

One particularly compelling application of meal templates is what I call the '80/20 approach' - having templates ready for about 80% of your regular meals while allowing flexibility for the remaining 20%. This balance provides structure where it's most beneficial while maintaining room for spontaneity and special occasions.

Remember that templates should serve as guidelines rather than rigid rules. They're tools to simplify your nutrition management, not restrictions that limit your food choices. As you become more comfortable with this system, you'll likely find yourself naturally developing new templates and variations that fit your preferences and lifestyle.

The goal of batch tracking and meal templates is to create a sustainable system that supports your nutrition goals while reducing the daily mental load of tracking. When implemented effectively, this approach can transform macro tracking from a time-consuming chore into a streamlined part of your daily routine, allowing you to maintain consistency without sacrificing flexibility or enjoyment in your food choices.

Tracking Challenges: Restaurant Meals, Social Events, and Travel

Maintaining consistent macro tracking when eating outside your routine presents unique challenges, but with the right strategies, you can stay on track without sacrificing social experiences or travel enjoyment. Through my years of coaching, I've developed practical approaches that help navigate these situations while maintaining a balanced relationship with food and nutrition goals.

When dining at restaurants, one of the most effective strategies is to research menus in advance. Most establishments now post their menus online, and many even provide nutritional information. This planning enables you to identify macro-friendly options before you sit down at the table. However, even without specific nutrition information, you can make educated estimates using some basic guidelines and visual cues.

Here are essential strategies for restaurant dining:

- Look for simple preparations (grilled, baked, steamed) over complex dishes

- Request sauces and dressings on the side

- Use hand portions to estimate serving sizes

- Choose dishes with clearly identifiable components

- Ask about preparation methods when unclear

Social events present their own set of challenges, often featuring buffet-style meals or passed appetizers that make tracking difficult. I worked with a client, Jennifer, who was struggling with maintaining her nutrition goals during wedding season. Together, we developed a strategy that we called the 'Social Event Success Plan.' Instead of trying to track every bite at events, she would adjust her meals earlier in the day to accommodate higher-calorie social functions and focus on protein-rich options when available.

Travel brings additional complexity to macro tracking, but it doesn't have to derail your nutrition goals. Whether you're traveling for business or pleasure, maintaining awareness of your macro intake is possible with some planning and flexible strategies. I learned this firsthand during a busy conference season where I was traveling weekly.

Here are proven strategies for travel nutrition management:

- Pack protein-rich snacks for travel days

- Research nearby restaurants and grocery stores at your destination

- Book accommodations with kitchen facilities when possible

- Maintain regular meal timing across time zones

- Focus on protein and vegetable portions when dining out

One efficient approach I've developed with clients is the 'anchor meal' strategy. This involves planning one main meal each day that hits specific macro targets, then building flexibility around that anchor point. For instance, if you know you're having dinner at a restaurant, you can plan your breakfast and lunch to provide adequate protein and control overall macro intake.

Remember that perfect tracking isn't the goal during these situations - it's about maintaining awareness and making informed choices. I teach my clients to focus on protein portions first, as this tends to be the most challenging macro to hit when dining out. Once protein is addressed, you can build the rest of your meal around it with appropriate portions of carbohydrates and fats.

When faced with unknown portions or recipes, use these visual estimation guidelines:

- A palm-sized portion equals about 20-30g of protein

- A cupped hand represents about 20-30g of carbohydrates

- A thumb-sized portion approximates 7-9g of fat

These measurements aren't exact, but they provide a reliable framework for estimation when precise tracking isn't possible. The goal is to maintain awareness without becoming overly restrictive or anxious about exact numbers.

One of my clients, Michael, a frequent business traveler, developed a simple system using photo logging during trips. He would photograph his meals and make quick notes about the main components, then do a more detailed macro estimation at the end of the day. This approach allowed him to maintain awareness of his intake without disrupting business meetings or client dinners.

For special occasions and celebrations, I recommend the '80/20 approach'- focus on hitting your macro targets 80% of the time, while allowing flexibility for the other 20%. This might mean choosing your most macro-friendly options for most meals, but enjoying unique dishes or desserts in moderate portions without guilt.

The key to success in all these situations is preparation and flexibility. Having strategies in place before encountering challenging situations helps maintain consistency while allowing for the enjoyment of social occasions and travel experiences. Remember, the goal of macro tracking isn't to restrict your life but to enhance it by making informed choices that support your health and fitness goals.

Building Sustainable Tracking Habits: Finding Your Balance

Building sustainable tracking habits is like developing any other life skill—it requires patience, practice, and personalization. Through my years of nutrition coaching, I've discovered that the key to long-term success isn't finding the perfect tracking system, but rather creating habits that naturally align with your lifestyle and preferences. The goal is to develop a relationship with tracking that enhances your life rather than complicating it.

When I first started working with Sarah, a busy teacher and mother of two, she was struggling to maintain consistent tracking habits. She would start each week with enthusiasm, meticulously logging every meal, only to abandon the practice by Wednesday when life became hectic. Together, we developed a simplified approach that focused on key meals and essential portion awareness rather than precise measurements for every ingredient. This 'minimum effective dose' of tracking helped her maintain awareness without feeling overwhelmed.

Here are fundamental principles for building sustainable tracking habits:

- Start small with tracking just one meal per day

- Focus on consistency over perfection

- Build tracking into existing daily routines

- Use the simplest practical method for your lifestyle

- Create backup plans for busy days

The key to sustainable tracking is finding your balance point—the level of detail and commitment that you can maintain long-term without feeling stressed or overwhelmed. This might involve using detailed tracking during meal prep days, while relying on portion estimation when eating out, or maintaining stricter monitoring during the week and allowing more flexibility on weekends.

One effective strategy I've developed with clients is the 'habit stacking' approach. This involves attaching tracking activities to existing daily habits. For instance, if you already have a morning coffee routine, use that time to plan and pre-log your day's meals. Or if you regularly review your calendar before bed, add a quick check of your macro totals to that routine.

Creating sustainable tracking habits also involves developing systems tailored to various life situations. I encourage clients to create what I call 'tracking templates' for multiple scenarios:

- Regular workday meals

- Weekend social events

- Travel days

- Restaurant dining

- Holiday celebrations

These templates provide structure while maintaining flexibility, allowing you to adapt your tracking approach based on circumstances without having to abandon it entirely. The goal is to develop habits that bend rather than break when life gets challenging.

Remember that sustainable tracking isn't about achieving perfect accuracy every day. It's about maintaining consistent awareness of your nutrition while allowing for the natural ebb and flow of life. Some days you might track every gram of food, while others might involve more estimation and general awareness. Both approaches can be valid parts of a sustainable tracking practice.

One particularly effective method I've found is what I call the 'awareness scale' approach. Instead of viewing tracking as an all-or-nothing practice, consider it a spectrum of awareness levels. On some days, you might be at level 5, tracking everything in detail. For others, you might be at level 2, simply ensuring you're meeting your protein targets and maintaining reasonable portion sizes. This flexibility helps prevent the common 'perfect or nothing' mindset that often leads to abandoning tracking habits altogether.

The journey to finding your tracking balance is personal and often involves some trial and error. What works perfectly for one person might be unsustainable for another. The key is to be honest with yourself about what you can realistically maintain while still moving toward your nutrition goals. Start with more structure than you think you need, then gradually adjust based on your experience and results.

Building sustainable tracking habits also means developing strategies for recovery when you get off track. Instead of viewing missed tracking days as failures, treat them as learning opportunities. What caused the disruption? How could you handle similar situations in the future? This problem-solving approach helps build resilience and adaptability in your tracking practice.

Remember that the ultimate goal of tracking isn't the tracking itself, but rather the awareness and understanding of your nutrition that tracking provides. As you develop sustainable habits, you'll likely find that some aspects of tracking become more intuitive. You may need less detailed tracking for your regular meals, while maintaining more structured tracking for new recipes or meals from restaurants. This evolution is a natural part of the process and often leads to a more sustainable long-term approach to nutrition management. As we conclude this chapter on calorie counting and tracking strategies, let's reflect on the key principles we've explored together. Through Sarah's journey from obsessive tracking to finding balance, we've seen how understanding calories can become an empowering tool rather than a source of stress. We've learned that successful tracking isn't about perfect precision, but rather about developing sustainable habits that fit into our real lives.

The digital tools, manual methods, and batch tracking strategies we've discussed provide a flexible framework for managing your nutrition. Whether you prefer the technological convenience of apps or the mindful practice of food journaling, the key is finding an approach that feels natural and sustainable for your lifestyle. Remember that tracking challenges, such as restaurant meals, social events, and travel, are not obstacles to be feared, but opportunities to practice adaptable strategies.

Perhaps most importantly, we've discovered that building sustainable tracking habits isn't about adhering to rigid rules, but about creating systems that are flexible yet resilient. The 'anchor meal' strategy, visual portion guides, and template-based approaches we've explored offer practical solutions for maintaining awareness without sacrificing enjoyment or flexibility in your food choices.

As you move forward with your nutrition journey, remember that awareness, not perfection, is your goal. Start small, be consistent, and allow your tracking practice to evolve as you become more comfortable with these concepts. Whether you're aiming for weight management, improved performance, or better overall health, the tools and strategies in this chapter can help you create a sustainable approach to calorie awareness that supports your long-term success.

In the next chapter, we'll build upon these foundational tracking skills as we explore how to personalize your macro ratios for your specific goals and body type. But for now, focus on implementing one or two tracking strategies that resonate with you. Remember, every successful nutrition journey begins with small, consistent steps toward better awareness and understanding of your food choices.

Chapter 5

The 28-Day Macro Revolution:
Your Complete Meal Planning Guide

Creating your perfect macro balance is like composing a symphony - each instrument must play its part in perfect harmony to make beautiful music. Just as every musician brings their unique touch to an orchestra, your body has specific nutritional needs that require a personalized approach to macro-nutrition. Like an intricate dance, each macronutrient plays its unique role in your body's performance, and finding the right balance becomes a profoundly personal journey. The art of macro-nutrition lies not in following rigid formulas, but in understanding how to adjust these ratios to support your individual needs, goals, and lifestyle patterns.

Think of your body as a finely tuned instrument that requires specific fuel combinations to perform at its best. Just as a car requires the right mixture of fuel and air to run efficiently, your body needs an optimal balance of proteins, carbohydrates, and fats to function correctly. This balance isn't static – it shifts in response to your activity level, goals, and even the changing seasons of your life.

When I first started, I worked with a client named Maya who was training for her first marathon while juggling a demanding career in software development. She had been following a generic high-carb diet plan she found online, but was constantly feeling fatigued and struggling with recovery. Together, we analyzed her unique needs - her training schedule, work hours, stress levels, and eating preferences. We discovered that her body responded better to a modified macro ratio with slightly higher fats and moderate carbs, rather than the standard runner's diet she'd been following. By creating a personalized formula that accounted for her specific lifestyle factors and the signals from her body, Maya not only completed her marathon but also did so while feeling energized and strong. This experience reinforced my belief that nutrition isn't about following someone else's formula - it's about discovering what works best for your unique body and lifestyle.

In this chapter, we'll explore how to create a personalized macro-nutrition formula that adapts to your body's needs while supporting your health and fitness goals. We'll dive into the science behind macro customization, but more importantly, we'll focus on practical strategies for finding your optimal balance. Whether you're an athlete looking to enhance your performance, a busy professional seeking to maintain energy throughout the day, or someone simply looking to improve your health, you'll discover how to fine-tune your macro ratios for maximum benefit.

Remember, the journey to finding your perfect macro balance is a process of discovery. It requires patience, observation, and a willingness to adjust as your body provides feedback. Let's begin this exploration together, unlocking the potential of personalized macro-nutrition to transform your relationship with food and optimize your well-being.

Weekly Meal Planning Templates: Building Your 28-Day Framework

Building a successful 28-day meal planning framework starts with understanding that effective planning isn't about rigid schedules – it's about creating flexible templates that adapt to your life while maintaining your macro goals. Think of these templates as your nutritional building blocks, enabling you to create balanced meals that align with your schedule, preferences, and macro targets.

Let me share a practical approach I developed while working with busy professionals. Instead of creating strict day-by-day meal plans that often fail when life gets unpredictable, we focus on building weekly templates that provide structure while maintaining flexibility. Start by dividing your week into key meal periods, such as breakfast, lunch, dinner, and snacks. For each period, create a collection of 3-4 macro-balanced meal options that you enjoy and can prepare quickly and easily.

For example, your breakfast template might include:

- **Option 1:** Greek yogurt parfait with berries and granola (balanced protein and carbs)

- **Option 2:** Egg white omelet with vegetables and toast (higher protein focus)

- **Option 3**: Overnight oats with protein powder and nuts (make-ahead friendly)

This approach allows you to mix and match meals while maintaining your macro targets. The key is to ensure that each option within your template fits your calculated macro needs while providing variety and flexibility.

When building your 28-day framework, think in weekly blocks rather than trying to plan an entire month at once. Each week becomes a manageable unit that you can adjust and refine as needed. I recommend creating four distinct weekly templates that you can rotate throughout the month. This rotation helps prevent meal fatigue while maintaining the structure necessary for consistent macro tracking.

One of the most effective strategies I've found is the '3-3-3' approach: plan three breakfast options, three lunch options, and three dinner templates that you can modify with different proteins or vegetables. This creates enough variety to prevent boredom while keeping your planning manageable. For instance, a dinner template might be:

- Protein + roasted vegetables + grain

- Protein + salad + starchy vegetable

- One-pan protein and vegetable stir-fry

The beauty of this system lies in its adaptability. Each template can be customized with different ingredients while maintaining similar macro ratios. A stir-fry template could feature chicken one week and tofu the next, with various vegetable combinations, yet still hit your target macros.

To make your 28-day framework truly sustainable, include planned flexibility. Designate specific meals or days where you'll eat out or enjoy social occasions. This might mean having two 'flex meals' per week where you focus on portion control rather than strict macro counting. Building this flexibility into your framework helps prevent the all-or-nothing mindset that often derails long-term success.

Remember to include a simple shopping template that aligns with your meal plans. Break your grocery list into categories:

- Proteins (meats, fish, legumes, dairy)

- Carbohydrates (grains, fruits, starchy vegetables)

- Healthy fats (oils, nuts, avocados)

- Vegetables and greens

This categorization helps ensure you always have the right ingredients on hand to meet your macro targets while making shopping more efficient. Keep this template on your phone or posted in your kitchen for easy reference.

As you move through your 28-day framework, use a simple tracking system to note which meals worked well and which need adjustment. This feedback loop helps you refine your templates over time, making them increasingly personalized to your preferences and lifestyle. The goal isn't perfection – it's creating a sustainable system that supports your macro-nutrition goals while fitting seamlessly into your life.

Remember, your 28-day framework should evolve with you. As your schedule changes, your fitness goals shift, or you discover new favorite meals, don't hesitate to update your templates. The most successful meal plans are those that grow and adapt with your needs while maintaining the fundamental structure that supports your macro targets.

Strategic Grocery Shopping and Meal Prep Optimization

Strategic grocery shopping and meal prep optimization are the cornerstones of successful macro-nutrition implementation. When I first started coaching clients in macro-nutrition, I noticed that even those with perfect macro calculations would struggle without a solid shopping and prep strategy. The key is to approach both activities with a system that maximizes efficiency while minimizing stress and food waste.

Let's start with strategic grocery shopping. The most effective approach I've found is to organize your shopping list according to your macro targets rather than traditional grocery store layouts. Create three main categories on your list:

- Protein sources (meats, fish, eggs, dairy, legumes)

- Carbohydrate sources (grains, fruits, starchy vegetables)

- Healthy fat sources (oils, nuts, seeds, avocados)

This macro-based organization helps ensure you're purchasing the right balance of foods to meet your targets. Add a fourth category for non-starchy vegetables and greens, which provide essential nutrients while having minimal impact on your macro calculations.

One of the most valuable lessons I've learned about grocery shopping for macro success is the importance of buying in practical quantities. For example, if your weekly meal plan calls for 24 ounces of chicken breast, don't buy the family-size pack that contains 48 ounces unless you plan to freeze the excess. This precision helps prevent food waste while keeping your macro planning accurate.

When it comes to meal prep optimization, the key is to think in terms of components rather than complete meals. This approach, which I call the 'macro building blocks' method, involves preparing essential ingredients that can be mixed and matched throughout the week. For instance:

- Batch cook 2-3 protein sources

- Prepare 2-3 complex carbohydrates

- Pre-portion healthy fats

- Wash and cut vegetables for easy access

This component-based system provides flexibility while maintaining macro accuracy. Instead of being locked into pre-made meals, you can assemble various combinations tailored to your daily needs and preferences.

Time management is crucial for successful meal prep. I recommend the '2-hour power prep' approach:

- First 30 minutes: Oven-roasted proteins

- Next 30 minutes: Grains and complex carbs

- Next 30 minutes: Vegetable prep

- Final 30 minutes: Portioning and storage

Proper storage is essential for maintaining food quality and ensuring your prep work translates into convenient meals. Invest in quality containers that are both portion-appropriate and stackable. Label everything with dates and basic macro information for quick reference.

One of my favorite preparation strategies is what I call the 'I-I-I method': prepare one protein source that can be served hot, one that can be served cold, and one that is versatile enough for either. This provides variety while maintaining efficiency. For example:

- Grilled chicken breast (hot)

- Tuna salad (cold)

- Hard-boiled eggs (either)

Remember to consider your schedule when planning your prep sessions. If you know you have a busy week ahead, focus on preparing items that require more time to cook, like roasted vegetables or grains. Quick-cooking items, such as eggs or fish, can often be prepared fresh with minimal time investment.

A common mistake I see is trying to prep everything at once. Instead, I recommend what I call 'strategic partial prep'- thoroughly preparing foods that store well for 4-5 days (such as grains and roasted vegetables) while only partially preparing items that are best when fresh (like salad greens or fish). This ensures you're not sacrificing food quality for convenience.

Finally, develop a system for tracking what you've prepped and when it needs to be used. A simple whiteboard on your refrigerator listing prepared items and their 'use-by' dates can help prevent waste and enable you to plan mid-week meals effectively. This level of organization may seem excessive at first, but it becomes second nature with practice, making it significantly easier to maintain your macro targets.

Remember, the goal of strategic shopping and meal prep isn't perfection – it's creating a sustainable system that supports your macro-nutrition goals while fitting into your lifestyle. Begin with these fundamental principles and adjust them according to your schedule, preferences, and experience. Over time, you'll develop a personalized approach that makes macro-nutrition feel effortless rather than overwhelming.

Flexible Meal Timing and Portion Control Strategies

The timing of your meals and control of portions are two of the most powerful yet flexible tools in your macro-nutrition arsenal. Rather than adhering to rigid eating schedules or measuring every morsel, successful macro-nutrition focuses on developing sustainable strategies that work with your natural hunger cues and daily routine. Think of meal timing as a rhythm rather than a strict schedule – it should flow naturally with your day while supporting your energy needs and macro goals.

One of the most effective approaches I've developed with clients is what I call the 'Flexible 4-4-4 Framework.' This strategy divides your day into three flexible four-hour eating windows, with a fourth window for overnight fasting. The beauty of this system lies in its adaptability – you can shift these windows based on your schedule while maintaining consistent intervals between meals.

For example, if you start your day at 7 AM, your windows might look like:

-   Morning Window (7 AM - 11 AM)

- Midday Window (11 AM - 3 PM)

- Evening Window (3 PM - 7 PM)

- Rest Window (7 PM - 7 AM)

Within each window, you have the flexibility to eat when hungry, ensuring you hit your macro targets through a combination of meals and snacks. This approach helps prevent the common pitfalls of both under-eating and overeating while maintaining steady energy levels throughout the day.

When it comes to portion control, I teach clients to use their hands as portable measuring tools. This system is remarkably accurate for macro portions while being infinitely portable:

- Your palm determines protein portions

- Your cupped hand measures carbohydrate servings

- Your thumb indicates fat portions

- Your fist estimates vegetable servings

This hand-based measurement system becomes particularly valuable when dining out or in situations where food scales aren't practical. It provides a reliable way to estimate portions while maintaining the social enjoyment of eating.

One of the most successful strategies I've implemented with clients is the 'Plate Building Method.' This approach focuses on visual portioning rather than exact measurements:

- Fill 1/3 of your plate with protein

- Cover 1/3 with complex carbohydrates

- Reserve 1/3 for vegetables

- Add thumb-sized portions of healthy fats

This visual approach makes portion control intuitive rather than mathematical, while still maintaining appropriate macro ratios. It's particularly effective when combined with the Flexible 4-4-4 Framework, as it allows you to adjust portion sizes based on your hunger levels within each eating window.

For those who prefer more structure, I recommend using what I call 'Anchor Meals' – pre-planned meals that hit specific macro targets, around which you can flex the rest of your daily intake. For instance, having a consistent breakfast that provides 25% of your daily protein needs gives you a reliable foundation while allowing flexibility for lunch and dinner.

Remember that portion control isn't about restriction – it's about understanding appropriate serving sizes that support your macro goals while satisfying your hunger. The key is finding a balance between structure and flexibility that works for your lifestyle. Start with these basic frameworks and adjust them based on your body's feedback and daily routine.

When implementing these strategies, pay attention to your body's natural hunger and fullness cues. The goal is to establish a sustainable eating pattern that supports your macro targets while integrating naturally into your daily life. This may involve adjusting your eating windows or portion sizes according to your activity level, stress levels, or sleep patterns.

One particularly effective tool is the 'Macro Buffer Zone' concept – allowing for a 5-10% variance in portion sizes while maintaining overall macro balance. This flexibility helps prevent the all-or-nothing mindset that often derails nutrition plans while ensuring you stay within range of your targets.

As you develop your personal approach to meal timing and portion control, remember that consistency matters more than perfection. Focus on strategies that you can maintain long-term, rather than rigid rules that may work in the short term but are unsustainable. The most successful macro-nutrition plans are those that become natural habits rather than constant conscious efforts.

Adapting Your Plan: Solutions for Common Challenges

Even with the best-laid plans, challenges in maintaining your macro-nutrition goals are inevitable. The key to long-term success isn't avoiding these challenges but developing effective strategies to navigate them. Through my years of coaching, I've encountered numerous common obstacles and helped clients develop practical solutions that maintain progress without sacrificing lifestyle flexibility.

One of the most frequent challenges I encounter is dealing with unexpected schedule changes. Whether it's a last-minute meeting that runs through lunch or an impromptu dinner invitation, these situations can throw off carefully planned macro targets. The solution lies in developing what I call 'macro contingency plans.' These are pre-planned strategies that help you stay on track when your routine gets disrupted.

For instance, I worked with a client named Isabella, a busy executive who frequently faced unexpected schedule changes. We developed a simple three-tier backup plan:

- **Tier 1:** Portable macro-balanced snacks kept in her office drawer

- **Tier 2:** A list of quick macro-friendly options at nearby restaurants

- **Tier 3:** Frozen pre-portioned meals at home for late workdays

Another common challenge is managing macro targets during periods of high stress. When stress levels rise, many people find their eating habits become erratic. The solution isn't to enforce stricter control but to build more flexibility into your plan. I recommend using the '80/20 approach' during these times – focus on hitting your macro targets 80% of the time while allowing 20% flexibility for less precise tracking.

Travel presents its own set of challenges for maintaining a balanced diet. Whether for business or pleasure, being away from your usual food environment can make tracking difficult. The key is to focus on protein targets first, as this macronutrient has the most significant impact on satiety and body composition. Once you've secured your protein source, fill in carbohydrates and fats based on available options.

Here's a practical strategy for travel adaptation:

- Research hotel amenities (mini-fridge, microwave) in advance

- Pack protein powder or bars for backup

- Scout nearby grocery stores and restaurants

- Focus on portion control when exact tracking isn't possible

Social events and holidays often present challenges to macro-nutrition plans. Rather than avoiding these occasions or stressing about exact measurements, I teach clients to use the 'bracket method.' This involves slightly reducing macro intake in the days leading up to and following an event to create flexibility for social occasions while maintaining weekly averages.

Another significant challenge is navigating plateau periods, where progress appears to stall. The solution isn't always to make dramatic changes to your macro targets. Instead, focus on these adjustment strategies:

- Fine-tune meal timing

- Adjust food choices while maintaining macro ratios

- Increase water intake and sleep quality

- Review tracking accuracy

For those struggling with consistency in tracking, I recommend the 'template method.' Create pre-tracked templates for your most frequently consumed meals and snacks, thereby reducing the daily mental load of logging everything. This approach makes it easier to maintain awareness of your macro intake without feeling overwhelmed by constant tracking.

Sometimes the challenge isn't about the food itself but about maintaining motivation. I encourage clients to develop non-scale victories and progress markers that extend beyond simply achieving macro targets. These might include:

- Improved energy levels

- Better sleep quality

- Enhanced workout performance

- Consistent hunger patterns

- Improved digestion

When facing emotional eating challenges, the solution isn't to rely solely on willpower. Instead, develop a 'macro pause practice' – take a moment to check in with yourself before emotional eating episodes. This doesn't mean you can't eat; it means making a conscious choice about how to adjust your remaining macro targets if you do.

Remember that adaptation doesn't mean perfection. The goal is to develop solutions that work most of the time while maintaining progress toward your goals. Each challenge you successfully navigate adds to your toolkit of strategies, making future obstacles easier to handle.

One particularly effective strategy I've developed is the 'reset routine' – a simple three-step process for getting back on track after any disruption:

1. Return to your baseline macro targets without compensation

2. Review what triggered the disruption

3. Refine your contingency plans based on what you learned

This approach helps prevent the typical cycle of over-restriction that follows periods of macroeconomic plan disruption. Instead, it builds resilience and adaptability into your nutrition strategy, making it more sustainable in the long term.

The key to successful macro-nutrition isn't avoiding challenges but developing the tools and mindset to navigate them effectively. Each obstacle becomes an opportunity to refine your approach and build a more sustainable nutrition practice. Remember, the most successful long-term plans are those that can bend without breaking, adapting to life's inevitable challenges while maintaining progress toward your goals.

Progress Tracking and Plan Adjustments Throughout the Month

Effective progress tracking is the compass that guides your macro-nutrition journey, helping you understand what's working and what needs adjustment. I've found that successful tracking isn't about obsessing over daily numbers, but rather about identifying patterns and making informed adjustments that support your goals.

The most effective approach to progress tracking combines both quantitative and qualitative measures. While the scale and body measurements provide numerical data, equally important are energy levels, sleep quality, and how your clothes fit. I recommend creating a simple weekly check-in routine that includes:

- Body measurements (weight, circumference measurements)

- Progress photos from consistent angles

- Energy level ratings throughout the day

- Sleep quality assessment

- Workout performance metrics

One of the most valuable tools I've developed with clients is the 'Weekly Wellness Grid' - a simple chart that tracks both numerical data and subjective feelings. This provides a more comprehensive picture of your progress than numbers alone can convey.

When it comes to making adjustments to your plan, the key is to avoid reactive changes based on short-term fluctuations. Instead, look for patterns over 2-3 weeks before making significant modifications to your macro targets. Slight variations in weight and measurements are normal and often reflect factors such as water retention, stress, or hormonal changes, rather than actual progress stalls.

I recommend using what I call the '3-2-1 Rule' for plan adjustments:

- 3 weeks of consistent tracking before significant changes

- 2 data points showing the same trend

- 1 adjustment at a time

This methodical approach helps prevent the common mistake of making too many changes simultaneously, which can make it challenging to identify what's working.

When adjustments are needed, start with small changes to your macro ratios rather than dramatic overhauls. A 5-10% adjustment in any macro category is usually sufficient to restart progress while maintaining the sustainability of your plan. For example, if you're not seeing desired results, you might:

- Increase protein by 5-10% while reducing carbohydrates proportionally

- Adjust meal timing while maintaining the same macro totals

- Modify food choices while keeping macro ratios constant

One particularly effective strategy I use with clients is the 'Macro Cycling' approach, where we intentionally vary macro intake throughout the month to prevent plateaus and maintain metabolic flexibility. This might involve incorporating higher-carbohydrate days around intense workouts or strategically timing higher-fat days for recovery.

Remember that progress isn't always linear. There will be weeks where measurements don't change, but other markers of progress improve. This is why tracking multiple variables is crucial. A client might see no change on the scale but report better energy levels, improved sleep quality, and stronger workout performance—all valuable indicators of progress. This tracking gives you a sense of control and understanding of your body's response to different nutritional approaches.

For women, it's essential to consider monthly hormonal cycles when tracking progress and making adjustments. I recommend using a tracking app or journal that allows you to note your current stage in your cycle, as this can significantly impact water retention, energy levels, and hunger signals.

When reviewing your monthly progress, look for these key indicators of successful macro balance:

- Stable energy levels throughout the day

- Consistent hunger patterns

- Good sleep quality

- Steady workout performance

- Positive mood and mental clarity

If you notice persistent plateaus despite consistent adherence to your plan, consider these adjustment strategies:

• Review portion sizes and tracking accuracy

• Assess sleep quality and stress management

• Evaluate workout intensity and recovery

• Consider food quality and nutrient density

The goal of progress tracking isn't to create another source of stress but to provide actionable insights that guide your journey. Use your tracking data as a tool for empowerment rather than judgment. Each data point, whether positive or negative, provides valuable information about how your body responds to different nutritional approaches.

Remember that sustainable progress often comes from small, consistent adjustments rather than dramatic changes. Trust the process, stay consistent with your tracking, and make informed adjustments based on the patterns you observe. Your body will tell you what it needs - the key is learning to listen and respond appropriately. As we conclude this chapter on mastering macro balance, remember that creating your personalized nutrition formula is a journey of self-discovery and adaptation. Like Maya's story demonstrated, success comes not from following generic guidelines, but from understanding and responding to your body's unique needs. Through careful observation, thoughtful adjustments, and consistent application of the principles we've covered, you can develop a sustainable approach to macro-nutrition that supports your goals while fitting seamlessly into your lifestyle.

The strategies we've explored—from flexible meal timing to strategic grocery shopping and meal prep optimization—provide a comprehensive toolkit for your macronutrition journey. Remember that the '3-3-3' approach to meal planning, the hand-portion measurement system, and the Flexible 4-4-4 Framework are not rigid rules but adaptable guidelines that you can modify to suit your needs. These tools, combined with consistent progress tracking and strategic plan adjustments, create a foundation for long-term success.

Perhaps most importantly, we've learned that mastering macro balance isn't about perfection - it's about progress and sustainability. The skills and knowledge you've gained in this chapter will serve as your compass, helping you navigate various situations while maintaining your nutritional goals. Whether you're dealing with unexpected schedule changes, travel challenges, or social events, you now have the tools to make informed decisions that support your macro targets without sacrificing flexibility or enjoyment.

As you move forward, remember that your macro-nutrition journey is uniquely yours. What works perfectly for one person may need adjustment for another. Trust in the process of self-discovery, stay patient with your progress, and remain open to adjusting your approach as your body provides feedback. Your perfect macro balance is out there - it's simply a matter of finding the right combination of strategies that work for you.

In the next chapter, we'll explore how to put these principles into practice through innovative tracking strategies, providing you with practical tools to monitor and maintain your macro balance effectively. For now, take a moment to reflect on the concepts we've covered and consider how you can begin implementing them in your daily routine. Remember, every step forward, no matter how small, brings you closer to your goals in mastering macro-nutrition.

Chapter 6

Flexible Macro Solutions:
Dining Out and Social Situations

Creating your perfect macro balance is like composing a symphony - each instrument must play its part in perfect harmony to make beautiful music. Just as every musician brings their unique touch to a performance, your body has its own specific needs that require a personalized approach to macro-nutrition. As we dive deeper into the world of customized nutrition, you'll discover that your body's unique needs extend far beyond basic calorie counting. Think of crafting your macro formula as fine-tuning a sophisticated instrument - each adjustment, no matter how small, contributes to the overall harmony of your nutritional symphony, just like how a skilled musician must understand both music theory and their instrument's specific characteristics, mastering your macro balance requires understanding both nutritional science and your body's response patterns.

This personalization journey isn't just about numbers - it's about creating a sustainable approach that honors your body's unique requirements while supporting your goals. Through years of working with diverse clients, I've observed how individual factors, such as metabolism, activity level, stress patterns, and even sleep quality, can significantly impact optimal macro ratios. These observations have shaped my approach to macro-nutrition, moving away from rigid formulas toward more adaptable frameworks that can evolve with your changing needs.

During one of my nutrition workshops, I met a client named Marcus who was frustrated with following generic macro recommendations. As a vegetarian marathon runner, he struggled to meet his protein needs while maintaining enough carbohydrates for his training. Together, we analyzed his unique situation - his plant-based dietary preferences, high activity level, and specific performance goals. We discovered that the standard macro ratios weren't serving his needs. By adjusting his protein sources to include more legumes and plant-based proteins, and carefully calibrating his carbohydrate intake to match his training schedule, we created a personalized formula that worked well for his lifestyle. Within weeks, Marcus reported improved energy levels during his long runs and better recovery between training sessions. His success story perfectly illustrates why personalization is crucial in macro-nutrition - what works for one person may not work for another. This experience reinforced my belief that the most effective nutrition plan is one that's tailored to your individual needs and lifestyle.

In this chapter, we'll explore the art and science of creating your personalized macro formula. You'll learn how to assess your individual needs, understand the factors that influence your optimal macro balance, and develop strategies for adjusting your ratios as your body and goals evolve. Whether you're an athlete fine-tuning your performance nutrition or someone seeking better energy and health, the principles you'll discover will help you create a sustainable approach to macro-nutrition that's uniquely yours.

Restaurant Menu Navigation: Decoding Dishes and Making Smart Choices

Navigating restaurant menus while maintaining your macro goals might seem daunting at first, but with the right strategies, it becomes second nature. I recall when I first started teaching macro-nutrition; one of my clients would avoid eating out altogether, missing out on meaningful social connections due to fear of derailing her progress. Together, we developed a systematic approach that transformed her restaurant experience from one of stress to one of confidence.

The first step in mastering restaurant menu navigation is understanding standard cooking methods and their impact on macros. Grilled, broiled, and steamed items typically have fewer added fats than fried or sautéed options. When you see terms like 'crispy,' 'breaded,' or 'crusted,' it usually indicates the presence of additional carbohydrates and fats. Terms like 'glazed' or 'teriyaki' often signal hidden sugars, while 'creamy' or 'rich' typically indicate a higher fat content.

Let's break down some practical strategies for making macro-friendly choices:

- Start by identifying the protein source and cooking method
- Look for dishes that separate components (like a grilled chicken breast with sides)

- Request sauces and dressings on the side to control portions

- Ask about substitutions for higher-carb sides

- Consider splitting more significant portions or taking some home

One effective technique I teach my clients is the 'plate mapping' method. Before your food arrives, mentally divide your plate into sections: half for vegetables, a quarter for lean protein, and a quarter for complex carbohydrates. This visual guide helps maintain proper macro ratios even when exact measurements aren't possible.

When I'm dining out with clients, I often demonstrate how to ask strategic questions about meal preparation. Instead of asking complicated questions about exact ingredients, focus on simple requests, such as 'How is the chicken prepared?' or 'Can I have the sauce on the side?' Most restaurants are happy to accommodate basic modifications that can significantly impact the macro content of your meal.

Another valuable strategy is pre-planning. Many restaurants now post their menus online, often with nutritional information. Taking a few minutes to review the menu before arriving can help you make informed choices without feeling rushed or pressured. I encourage my clients to identify 2-3 suitable options before arriving, which helps prevent impulsive ordering decisions.

Remember that perfect macro tracking isn't always possible when dining out, and that's okay. The goal is to make the best choices available while enjoying the social aspect of dining. I teach my clients to focus on portion control and food quality rather than getting caught up in exact measurements. A helpful technique is to use your hand as a measuring tool: your palm for protein portions, your cupped hand for carbohydrates, and your thumb for fats.

One convenient approach I've developed with clients is what I call the 'macro balancing' technique. If you know you'll be dining out for dinner, adjust your earlier meals that day to accommodate a restaurant meal that might be higher in specific macros. This flexibility allows you to maintain your overall macro goals while enjoying dining out experiences.

When faced with limited menu options, focus on making the best possible choices rather than perfect ones. For example, if a salad comes with breaded chicken, request grilled chicken instead. If a dish comes with french fries, ask to substitute them with steamed vegetables or a side salad. These minor adjustments can significantly impact the macro composition of your meal while still allowing you to enjoy dining out.

Portion Size Estimation: Visual Tools and Practical Techniques

Understanding portion sizes without constantly measuring your food is a crucial skill for sustainable macro-nutrition success. When I first started teaching portion control, I noticed many clients becoming overwhelmed by the need to weigh and measure everything they ate. This led me to develop a practical system of visual tools that anyone can use to estimate portions, whether at home or dining out, accurately.

One of the most effective methods I've found is using your hands as portable measuring tools. Your palm can measure protein portions (about 3-4 ounces), your cupped hand estimates carbohydrate servings, your thumb approximates fat portions, and your fist represents a cup of vegetables. This system is particularly valuable because it's proportional to your body size, naturally accounting for different portion needs among individuals.

Let me share a practical example that transformed how one of my clients approached portion estimation. Sarah, a busy executive, was struggling with portion control during her workday lunches. Together, we created a visual reference guide using common objects she always had access to:

- A deck of cards = 3 ounces of protein

- A tennis ball = 1/2 cup of complex carbohydrates

- A golf ball = 2 tablespoons of healthy fats

- A baseball = 1 cup of vegetables

- A pair of dice = 1 ounce of cheese

Beyond hand measurements and everyday objects, another powerful technique is the plate method. I teach clients to mentally divide their plate into sections: half for vegetables, a quarter for lean protein, and a quarter for complex carbohydrates. This visual approach helps maintain proper macro ratios without requiring precise measurements.

Photography can also be a valuable tool for portion training. I encourage clients to take photos of properly measured portions of their commonly eaten foods, creating a personal visual reference library. This technique helped one of my clients, Michael, develop an almost intuitive sense of portion sizes after just a few weeks of practice.

When eating out, where measuring tools aren't available, visual estimation becomes even more crucial. I teach a technique I call 'restaurant reconnaissance,' which involves using menu descriptions and visual cues to estimate portion sizes. For example, most restaurants serve protein portions that are about the size of a smartphone or deck of cards, while a side of rice or pasta is typically about the size of a tennis ball.

It's important to remember that portion estimation is a skill that improves with practice. I recommend periodically checking your estimates against actual measurements to maintain accuracy. This 'calibration process' helps refine your visual estimation skills over time.

One particularly effective exercise I use with clients is the 'portion practice plate' technique. Set up a meal with your usual portions, estimate the amounts using visual tools, and then measure them accurately. This feedback loop helps train your eye to naturally recognize proper portion sizes.

Remember that portion estimation isn't about perfect precision - it's about consistency and awareness. Even if your estimates are off by small amounts, maintaining consistent portions will help you achieve more reliable results than alternating between very large and very small servings.

To build confidence in your estimation skills, start with foods you eat regularly. Create a reference sheet with photos or drawings of your common meals, noting the proper portions alongside your visual cues. This personalized guide becomes an invaluable tool for maintaining portion awareness without the need for constant measuring.

Through years of teaching these techniques, I've found that most people can become quite accurate at portion estimation within a few weeks of consistent practice. The key is to start simple, focus on your most frequently consumed foods, and gradually expand your estimation skills to include a wider variety of items.

Social Event Strategies: Handling Pressure and Managing Special Occasions

Special occasions and social events often present unique challenges for maintaining macro-nutrition goals. The combination of festive food, social pressure, and disrupted routines can make it tempting to abandon your nutritional awareness altogether. However, with thoughtful preparation and the right mindset, you can navigate these situations while staying aligned with your goals and thoroughly enjoying the celebration.

I recall working with a client, Jennifer, who was preparing for her best friend's wedding weekend, complete with a rehearsal dinner, wedding reception, and farewell brunch. She was worried about maintaining her nutrition progress during the celebrations without appearing antisocial or drawing attention to her food choices. Together, we developed strategies that allowed her to fully participate in the festivities while staying mindful of her macro goals.

- Here are some proven strategies for managing special occasions:

- Eat a protein-rich snack before events to avoid arriving overly hungry

- Survey the entire buffet or menu before making selections

- Choose your indulgences mindfully - focus on special items you genuinely enjoy

- Practice the 'one-plate rule' at buffets to avoid mindless grazing

- Stay hydrated with water between alcoholic beverages

One of the most challenging aspects of social events is managing well-meaning pressure from friends and family. I teach my clients the art of graceful deflection - simple phrases like 'I'm pacing myself' or 'I'm saving room for dessert' can help avoid lengthy discussions about food choices while maintaining social harmony.

When it comes to holiday seasons or extended celebration periods, I recommend using what I call the '80/20 approach.' Focus on maintaining your usual macro awareness for 80% of your meals, allowing for more flexibility during special occasions that make up the other 20%. This balance helps prevent the all-or-nothing mindset that often leads to abandoning nutrition goals altogether.

Another effective strategy is what I call 'pre-event planning.' Before attending a social gathering, take a few minutes to visualize the event and plan your approach. Consider factors like timing, available food options, and potential challenges. This mental preparation helps you make conscious choices rather than reactive decisions in the moment.

I worked with a client, Michael, who struggled with business dinners until we developed his 'social event toolkit.' This included strategies such as reviewing restaurant menus in advance, identifying macro-friendly options, and practicing polite ways to decline excessive food offerings from colleagues. Within months, he was confidently navigating business meals while maintaining his nutrition goals.

Remember that perfect macro adherence isn't the goal during special occasions. Instead, focus on maintaining awareness and making conscious choices. I encourage clients to enjoy traditional family dishes or celebration foods in moderate portions, then return to their usual eating patterns for the next meal. This approach helps prevent the guilt and anxiety that often accompany special occasions.

For multi-day events or holiday seasons, implement what I call the 'bookmark strategy.' Treat the days before and after special occasions as 'bookmarks' where you maintain your usual macro awareness. This helps create a natural boundary around celebration times, preventing one day of flexibility from turning into weeks of unstructured eating.

One particularly effective technique for managing social pressure is to take on the role of either a host or a contributor. By bringing a macro-friendly dish to share or hosting events where you can control some of the food options, you ensure there are always choices that align with your goals while contributing positively to the celebration.

Lastly, remember that social connections and celebrations are essential components of a healthy lifestyle. The goal isn't to achieve perfect macro ratios during these times, but rather to find a balance that allows you to maintain your overall progress while fully participating in life's special moments. With practice, these strategies become natural habits that help you navigate any social situation with confidence and ease.

Pre-planning and Post-event Macro Adjustments

Successfully managing special events while maintaining your macro goals requires both thoughtful pre-planning and strategic post-event adjustments. Through my years of nutrition coaching, I've developed a systematic approach that helps clients navigate celebrations and special occasions without derailing their progress or missing out on enjoyable experiences.

Pre-event planning begins with understanding the context of your event. I teach clients to consider factors like timing, duration, and available food options. For instance, if you're attending an evening wedding reception, you can adjust your earlier meals that day to accommodate the celebration. This might mean increasing protein and vegetable intake during breakfast and lunch while reducing carbohydrates and fats, saving those macro allowances for the evening event.

One of my clients, Lisa, mastered this approach during her company's annual conference week. She would start each day with a protein-rich breakfast and pack macro-balanced snacks for between sessions. This preparation enabled her to participate in networking dinners while maintaining a balanced overall macro intake throughout the week.

Here are key pre-event strategies that have proven successful:

- Review your total daily macro targets and allocate portions for the event

- Eat a balanced meal 2-3 hours before the event to avoid arriving overly hungry

- Pack portable protein options for long events

- Plan your hydration strategy, especially if alcohol will be involved

- Identify potential macro-friendly choices at the venue in advance

Equally important is having a post-event adjustment strategy in place. The goal isn't to 'compensate' for enjoyment, but rather to ease back into your regular macro routine smoothly. I recommend what I call the 'gradual reset approach' - instead of drastically cutting calories the next day, focus on returning to standard portion sizes and macro ratios over the following 2-3 meals.

Post-event adjustments should focus on these key areas:

- Prioritize protein and fiber-rich vegetables in your next few meals

- Increase water intake to support digestion and hydration

- Return to regular meal timing and portion sizes

- Focus on nutrient-dense foods rather than restriction

- Resume regular tracking without guilt about the special event

One particularly effective technique I've developed is the 'macro averaging' approach. Rather than viewing each day in isolation, consider your macro intake across a broader timeframe, such as a week. This perspective helps maintain flexibility for special events while keeping your overall nutrition on track.

I worked with a client, Marcus, who frequently attended business dinners. We created a weekly macro plan that allocated slightly higher allowances for dinner events, balanced by more structured meals on other days. This strategy allowed him to maintain his progress while confidently participating in essential business functions.

Remember that successful macro management isn't about perfect adherence every single day. It's about creating sustainable patterns that accommodate both your nutrition goals and life's special moments. The key is having strategic approaches for both pre-planning and post-event adjustments that help you maintain overall consistency.

When implementing post-event adjustments, avoid the common pitfall of overcompensation. I've seen many people attempt to 'make up for' an indulgent event by severely restricting their intake the next day. This approach often backfires, leading to energy crashes and an increased risk of overeating. Instead, focus on returning to your regular, balanced macro intake pattern.

One helpful tool I recommend is keeping a 'flexible events calendar.' By noting upcoming special occasions, you can better plan your macro adjustments and maintain a balanced approach to nutrition, allowing you to enjoy life's celebrations fully. This proactive strategy helps prevent the stress and anxiety that often accompany unexpected dietary changes.

Building a Flexible Mindset: Balance Over Perfection

Developing a flexible mindset around macro-nutrition is essential for long-term success. Throughout my years of coaching, I've observed that clients who embrace flexibility while maintaining awareness consistently achieve better results than those who strive for perfection. This journey isn't about following your macro targets with military precision - it's about creating a sustainable approach that adapts to your life's natural ebbs and flows.

I recall working with Rachel, a perfectionist who meticulously tracked every gram of food and became anxious when she couldn't measure her portions precisely. Her rigid approach was creating stress and making it difficult to maintain her nutrition goals in real-world situations. Together, we developed what I call the '85/15 approach' - focusing on consistent, mindful choices 85% of the time, while allowing flexibility for the remaining 15%. This simple shift in perspective transformed her relationship with food and her approach to macro tracking.

Building a flexible mindset begins with understanding that consistency is more important than perfection. Think of your macro goals as a target range rather than exact numbers. Just as an archer might aim for the bullseye but still score points hitting the surrounding rings, you can make progress while allowing for natural variation in your daily macro intake.

Here are the key principles for developing macro flexibility:

- Focus on weekly averages rather than daily perfection

- Allow for natural variation in hunger and portion sizes

- Practice adaptable tracking methods for different situations

- Develop strategies for handling unexpected food scenarios

- Learn to trust your body's signals while maintaining awareness

One effective technique I teach clients is the 'macro banking' approach. If you know you'll be having dinner at a restaurant where precise tracking is challenging, you can adjust your earlier meals to accommodate more flexibility later. This isn't about restriction, but rather about thoughtful planning that allows for both structure and spontaneity.

Another client, Michael, struggled with all-or-nothing thinking around his macro goals. When he couldn't hit his exact targets, he would abandon tracking altogether, leading to cycles of strict adherence followed by complete disconnection from his nutrition awareness. We worked on developing what I call 'flexible precision' - using exact measurements when practical, while having reliable estimation methods for other situations.

Remember that your body doesn't operate on a 24-hour reset button. Examining your macro intake over a broader timeframe, such as a week, offers more flexibility while maintaining overall consistency. This perspective helps prevent the stress and anxiety that often accompany rigid tracking approaches.

I encourage clients to practice 'mindful flexibility' by asking themselves these questions when facing food decisions:

- Will this choice support my overall goals?

- Can I make minor adjustments to improve the macro balance?

- How can I enjoy this situation while maintaining awareness?

- What's the most practical approach at this moment?

Developing a flexible mindset also means learning to navigate setbacks without viewing them as failures. Instead of seeing a day of off-target macros as a disaster, treat it as valuable feedback that helps you refine your approach. This resilient perspective builds confidence in your ability to maintain long-term nutrition awareness.

One particularly effective strategy is what I refer to as the 'macro hierarchy.' When faced with situations where perfect tracking isn't practical, focus first on protein targets, then on overall portion size, and finally on the balance of carbohydrates and fats. This prioritization helps maintain the most important aspects of your nutrition while allowing flexibility in other areas.

The goal of macro-nutrition isn't to create a perfect scorecard of hitting exact numbers every day. Instead, think of it as developing a sustainable lifestyle that supports your health and fitness goals while accommodating the natural variations of daily life. With practice, this flexible mindset becomes second nature, enabling you to maintain awareness without the stress of striving for perfection. As we conclude this chapter on personalizing your macro-nutrition approach, remember that creating your perfect macro balance is an evolving journey rather than a fixed destination. Throughout the chapter, we've explored how different body types respond uniquely to various macro ratios, just as Marcus discovered when adapting his vegetarian marathon training diet. Your optimal macro formula will likely shift as your goals, activity levels, and lifestyle change over time.

The key principles we've covered—ranging from understanding menu navigation to mastering portion estimation and handling social situations—all work together to create a sustainable approach to macronutrition. These tools aren't meant to restrict your life but rather to enhance it by providing the flexibility and awareness needed for long-term success. The pre-planning and post-event adjustment strategies we discussed demonstrate how macro awareness can coexist with life's celebrations and memorable moments.

Remember the story of Lisa, who transformed her relationship with restaurant dining from stress to confidence through practical portion estimation techniques. Her experience demonstrates that with the right tools and mindset, one can maintain one's macro awareness in any situation. The flexible mindset we explored isn't about pursuing perfection - it's about creating sustainable habits that adapt to your life's natural rhythms.

As you move forward with your macro-nutrition journey, focus on progress over perfection. Use the hand measurement techniques, visual estimation tools, and social event strategies we've discussed to build confidence in your ability to make informed choices. Whether you're dining out, attending celebrations, or managing busy workdays, you now have a toolbox of practical strategies to help you maintain your macro balance while fully participating in life's experiences.

In the next chapter, we'll explore practical tracking methods that make macro monitoring manageable in real-world situations. For now, take the time to practice the personalization techniques we've covered. Start with small adjustments, observe how your body responds, and gradually refine your approach. Remember, the most effective nutrition plan is one that you can maintain consistently while enjoying the journey toward your health and fitness goals.

Chapter 7

——————‸——————

Fine-Tuning Your Macro Type: Adapting Macros for Different Body Types and Goals

In today's digital age, tracking your nutrition doesn't require carrying around a notebook and calculator - technology has transformed how we monitor our food intake and understand our eating habits. Whether you prefer apps, spreadsheets, or simple paper journals, finding the proper tracking method can make the difference between sustainable success and frustrated abandonment of your nutrition goals. The evolution of nutrition tracking, from pen-and-paper to sophisticated mobile apps, has transformed how we approach our dietary goals; however, finding the right method amidst these options remains a personal journey. Like any skill worth mastering, effective tracking requires a balance of knowledge, practice, and the right tools for your lifestyle.

Whether you're new to macro tracking or looking to refine your approach, this chapter will equip you with practical strategies that work in real-world situations. We'll explore various tracking methods, from high-tech solutions to simple visual guides, helping you find an approach that fits seamlessly into your daily routine without becoming a source of stress or obsession.

During a weekend nutrition workshop, I encountered a client named Tom who worked as a traveling sales representative. He was struggling to maintain consistent macro tracking due to his frequent business trips and client dinners. His current system of trying to weigh every food item was causing stress and making him avoid social situations. Together, we developed a practical approach using hand measurements and photo logging. I taught him how to measure protein portions with his palm, carbohydrates with his cupped hand, and fats with his thumb. We also found a user-friendly app that allowed quick visual logging.

Six months later, Tom shared how this simplified system had transformed his relationship with food tracking. He was hitting his macro goals while confidently navigating business dinners and travel days. His success story perfectly illustrates how finding the right tracking strategy can transform what seems like an overwhelming task into a manageable and even enjoyable part of daily life.

In this chapter, we'll explore proven tracking techniques that can adapt to various lifestyles, from busy professionals to home-based parents. You'll learn how to choose the right tools, develop sustainable habits, and overcome common tracking challenges. Most importantly, you'll discover how to maintain awareness of your nutrition goals without letting tracking dominate your daily life.

Remember, the goal isn't to track every morsel with perfect precision, but rather to develop a practical system that helps you consistently make informed food choices. Whether you prefer digital tools or simple visual guides, we'll help you find and refine your perfect tracking strategy.

Understanding Different Body Types and Their Macro Needs

Just as no two fingerprints are exactly alike, our bodies respond differently to various macro ratios based on our unique body composition and metabolic characteristics. Understanding your body type is crucial for optimizing your macronutrient approach and achieving your health and fitness goals effectively.

There are three primary body types: ectomorph, mesomorph, and endomorph, each with distinct characteristics that influence how they process and utilize macronutrients. While most people are a blend of these types, identifying your dominant characteristics can help guide your macro-nutrition strategy.

Ectomorphs typically have a lean, long-limbed build with fast metabolism. These "hard gainers" often struggle to maintain weight and muscle mass. For ectomorphs, a higher carbohydrate intake (around 50-55% of total calories) can support their naturally high metabolic rate, while maintaining moderate protein (20-25%) and lower fat (25-30%) ratios. This macro distribution helps fuel their active metabolism while supporting muscle maintenance and repair.

Mesomorphs tend to have an athletic, muscular build and respond well to exercise. Their bodies efficiently build muscle and maintain a relatively stable body composition. A balanced macro approach often works best for mesomorphs, with roughly equal proportions of proteins and carbohydrates (35-40% each) and moderate fat intake (25-30%). This distribution supports their natural tendency to build and maintain muscle while providing steady energy.

Endomorphs typically have a larger bone structure and higher tendencies for body fat storage. They often face challenges with weight management and may be more sensitive to carbohydrates. For endomorphs, a higher protein intake (35-40% of calories) combined with moderate fat (30-35%) and lower carbohydrate (25-30%) ratios often proves most effective. This distribution helps manage insulin sensitivity while supporting satiety and muscle preservation.

During my years of nutrition and wellness coaching, I worked with a client named Ariana who perfectly illustrated the importance of body type-specific macro ratios. As an endomorph who had been following a high-carbohydrate diet designed for ectomorphs, she struggled with constant hunger and energy crashes. When we adjusted her macros to align with her body type, increasing protein and healthy fats while moderating carbohydrates, she experienced improved energy levels and better progress toward her goals.

However, it's essential to remember that these guidelines are starting points, not rigid rules. Your optimal macro ratio may vary based on factors such as activity level, age, hormonal balance, and specific health goals. Regular monitoring and adjustment of your macro intake, based on your body's response, is key to long-term success.

To find your optimal macro balance, start with the general guidelines for your body type and then:

- Monitor your energy levels throughout the day

- Track your hunger and satiety signals

- Observe your exercise performance and recovery

- Note any changes in body composition

- Pay attention to sleep quality and mood

These indicators will help you fine-tune your macro ratios to find what works best for your unique physiology. Remember that your needs may change over time as your body composition, activity level, or goals evolve.

The key to success is viewing your body type not as a limitation but as a guide to understanding your nutritional needs. By aligning your macro intake with your natural physiology, you can create a more effective and sustainable approach to reaching your health and fitness goals.

Goal-Specific Macro Adjustments: From Fat Loss to Muscle Gain

Understanding how to adjust your macronutrient ratios based on specific fitness goals is crucial for achieving optimal results. Whether you're aiming to lose fat, build muscle, or maintain your current composition, your macro needs will vary significantly. Let's explore how to tailor your macro intake for different objectives while maintaining a balanced and sustainable approach.

For fat loss goals, creating a moderate caloric deficit while preserving muscle mass is key. This typically involves:

- Higher protein intake (30-35% of total calories)

- Moderate fat intake (25-30% of total calories)

- Lower, but adequate carbohydrates (35-40% of total calories)

This distribution helps maintain satiety, preserve lean muscle mass, and provide enough energy for daily activities and workouts. The higher protein intake is particularly important during fat loss phases to prevent muscle breakdown while in a caloric deficit.

For muscle gain objectives, the focus shifts to providing adequate nutrients for growth and recovery while maintaining a slight caloric surplus. A typical macro distribution might include:

- Moderate to high protein (25-30% of total calories)

- Moderate fat (20-25% of total calories)

- Higher carbohydrates (45-55% of total calories)

Increased carbohydrate intake supports intense training sessions and helps fuel muscle growth, while protein remains crucial for muscle tissue repair and development.

During my years as a nutrition coach, I worked with a client named James who perfectly illustrated the importance of goal-specific macro adjustments. He initially came to me frustrated after months of trying to build muscle while following a low-carb, high-protein diet that had previously helped him lose fat. By adjusting his macros to include more carbohydrates around his training sessions and maintaining moderate protein levels, his energy and strength in the gym improved significantly, leading to better muscle gains.

For maintenance phases, finding a balanced approach that supports your activity level while maintaining body composition is essential. This often involves:

- Moderate protein (25-30% of total calories)

- Moderate fat (25-30% of total calories)

- Moderate carbohydrates (40-50% of total calories)

Remember that these ratios serve as starting points and should be adjusted according to individual responses and preferences. Factors to consider when fine-tuning your macro ratios include:

- Training intensity and frequency

- Daily activity level

- Personal food preferences

- Digestive tolerance

- Recovery needs

The key to successful macro adjustments is making gradual changes and monitoring your body's response to them. Start with minor adjustments of 5-10% in any macro category and observe the effects over 2-3 weeks before making further changes. This methodical approach helps identify what works best for your body while maintaining sustainable progress toward your goals.

When transitioning between different goals, it's essential to make changes gradually. For example, when transitioning from a fat loss phase to a muscle-building phase, gradually increase your calories and adjust your macros over several weeks, rather than making dramatic changes all at once. This approach helps your body adapt and minimizes unwanted fat gain or metabolic disruption.

Regardless of your specific goal, maintaining consistent protein intake across different phases helps preserve muscle mass and supports recovery. The main variables to adjust are typically your carbohydrate and fat ratios, which can be modified based on your activity level and how your body responds to different macro distributions.

Remember that successful macro adjustment isn't just about hitting specific numbers - it's about finding a sustainable approach that supports your goals while fitting into your lifestyle. The ideal macro ratio is one that you can consistently maintain while making progress toward your objectives.

Age and Gender Considerations in Macro Distribution

As we progress through various life stages, our nutritional needs change, necessitating thoughtful adjustments to our macronutrient distribution. Understanding how age and gender influence our macro requirements is crucial for maintaining optimal health and achieving our fitness goals effectively.

Women typically require different macro distributions compared to men due to hormonal differences and variations in body composition. Women usually require a higher percentage of essential fats (approximately 25-35% of total calories) to support hormonal function and reproductive health. Protein needs typically range from 0.8 to 1.2 grams per pound of body weight, while carbohydrate requirements vary based on activity level and individual response.

Men, on the other hand, typically benefit from higher protein intake (around 1.0-1.5g per pound of body weight) to support greater muscle mass and higher metabolic demands. Their carbohydrate needs often align with their activity levels, while fat intake can be moderately lower than women's requirements, typically ranging from 20% to 30% of total calories.

During my nutrition practice, I worked with a couple, Sarah and Mike, who highlighted these differences perfectly. Despite following the same workout routine, their bodies responded differently to various macro distributions. Sarah struggled with energy levels and hormonal balance until we increased her healthy fat intake to 30% of her total calories. Meanwhile, Mike's recovery and muscle maintenance improved significantly when we adjusted his protein intake to the higher end of the range.

Age also plays a crucial role in determining optimal macro distribution. As we age, our protein needs typically increase to help maintain muscle mass and support healthy aging. For adults over 50, protein requirements typically range from 1.2 to 1.6 grams per pound of body weight, with a focus on evenly distributing protein intake throughout the day.

Consider these age-specific considerations when adjusting your macros:

- Young Adults (20-35): Focus on balanced ratios with adequate protein for muscle development and maintenance

- Middle Age (35-50): Gradually increase protein while maintaining carbohydrates based on activity level

- Older Adults (50+): Higher protein needs with moderate carbohydrates and adequate healthy fats

- Post-Menopausal Women: Increased protein needs with emphasis on healthy fats for hormonal support

Hormonal changes throughout life also influence macro needs. For women, menstrual cycles can affect carbohydrate utilization and cravings. During the luteal phase, many women benefit from slightly higher carbohydrate intake to support energy levels and mood regulation. Similarly, during menopause, women often need to adjust their macronutrient ratios to account for changes in hormonal profiles and metabolism.

I recall working with Linda, a 55-year-old client who was experiencing menopause. Her previous macro distribution, which had worked well for years, suddenly seemed ineffective. By increasing her protein intake to 1.4g per pound of body weight and adjusting her carbohydrate timing around her workouts, we helped her maintain her lean mass and energy levels during this transitional period.

Regardless of age or gender, it's essential to remember that these guidelines are starting points. Individual factors such as activity level, health status, and specific goals should always influence your final macro distribution. Regular monitoring and adjustment based on your body's response remains key to finding your optimal balance.

When adjusting your macros based on age and gender, consider these practical strategies:

- Monitor energy levels and recovery capacity

- Pay attention to hunger and satiety signals

- Track strength and endurance during workouts

- Observe changes in body composition

- Note mood and sleep quality

These indicators can help you fine-tune your macro ratios to better suit your individual needs, while also taking into account age and gender-specific considerations. Remember that nutrition is a journey that evolves with you, and your macro needs will continue to change throughout different life stages.

The key to success is viewing these age and gender considerations not as limitations but as guidelines for optimizing your nutrition approach. By understanding and adapting to your body's changing needs, you can maintain a sustainable and effective nutrition strategy throughout your life.

Activity Level Impact on Macro Requirements

Your activity level plays a crucial role in determining your macro requirements, as physical activity significantly impacts how your body utilizes and processes nutrients. Understanding how to adjust your macros based on your activity level is essential for optimizing performance, recovery, and overall health.

Physical activity increases your body's demand for energy and specific nutrients, particularly carbohydrates for fuel and protein for muscle repair and growth. The more active you are, the higher your caloric and macro needs become. However, these increases aren't linear - they depend on the type, intensity, and duration of your activities.

Let's break down macro requirements for different activity levels:

- Sedentary (Little to no exercise)

- Light Activity (1-3 days/week of exercise)

- Moderate Activity (3-5 days/week of exercise)

- Very Active (6-7 days/week of exercise)

- Highly Active (Multiple daily training sessions)

For sedentary individuals, macro needs are relatively modest. A typical distribution might include:

- Protein: 0.8-1.0g per pound of body weight

- Carbohydrates: 30-40% of total calories

- Fats: 25-35% of total calories

As activity levels increase, carbohydrate and protein needs typically rise to support performance and recovery. For example, a moderately active person might require:

- Protein: 1.0-1.2g per pound of body weight

- Carbohydrates: 40-50% of total calories

- Fats: 25-30% of total calories

During my years as a nutrition coach, I worked with a client named Rachel who perfectly illustrated the importance of activity-based macro adjustments. As a former sedentary office worker who began training for a half-marathon, her initial macro distribution wasn't supporting her new level of activity. She frequently felt fatigued during her longer runs and struggled with recovery. By increasing her carbohydrate intake around her training sessions and slightly boosting her overall protein intake, her energy levels stabilized and her recovery improved significantly.

For very active individuals, particularly those engaging in intense training, macro needs increase substantially:

- Protein: 1.2-1.5g per pound of body weight

- Carbohydrates: 50-60% of total calories

- Fats: 20-25% of total calories

The timing of your macro intake becomes increasingly important as activity levels rise. Consider these key principles for active individuals:

• Pre-workout nutrition should focus on easily digestible carbohydrates

• Post-workout meals should combine protein and carbohydrates for recovery

• Fats should be consumed further from training sessions to optimize performance

When adjusting your macros based on activity level, pay attention to these indicators:

- Energy levels during workouts

- Recovery between sessions

- Muscle soreness and fatigue

- Performance progress

- Overall mood and well-being

Remember that activity level isn't static - it can change weekly or even daily. Your macro needs should be flexible enough to accommodate these variations. For example, you might increase carbohydrates on training days and reduce them slightly on rest days while keeping protein relatively constant.

I often recommend creating two different macro targets: one for training days and one for rest days. This approach allows for better nutrient periodization while maintaining overall balance. The difference typically involves adjusting carbohydrate intake while keeping protein and fat relatively stable.

For example, a moderately active person might adjust their macros as follows:

Training Days:

- Higher carbohydrate intake (45-55% of calories)

- Moderate protein (25-30% of calories)

- Lower fat (20-25% of calories)

Rest Days:

- Lower carbohydrate intake (35-45% of calories)

- Moderate protein (25-30% of calories)

- Higher fat (25-35% of calories)

The key to successful activity-based macro adjustment is listening to your body's signals while maintaining consistency with your overall nutrition plan. Start with the baseline recommendations for your activity level, then make small adjustments based on your performance, recovery, and energy levels.

Remember that these guidelines serve as starting points; your individual needs may vary based on factors such as body composition, training goals, and the specific demands of your chosen activities. Regular monitoring and adjustment of your macro intake, based on your body's response and performance feedback, will help you optimize your nutrition for your specific activity level.

Progress Monitoring and Macro Fine-Tuning Strategies

Successful macro-nutrition isn't just about setting initial targets - it's about monitoring your progress and making strategic adjustments based on your body's response. Like a skilled navigator who constantly checks their coordinates and adjusts their course, you need to regularly assess your progress and fine-tune your macro intake for optimal results.

The key to effective progress monitoring lies in tracking both quantitative and qualitative indicators. While the scale can provide some insight, it shouldn't be your only measure of progress. Consider tracking these key indicators:

- Body measurements (waist, hips, chest, arms)

- Energy levels throughout the day

- Workout performance and recovery

- Sleep quality

- Hunger and satiety signals

- Mood and mental clarity

During my nutrition coaching practice, I worked with a client named Jamie who taught me a valuable lesson about the importance of comprehensive progress monitoring. Initially focused solely on the scale, Jamie became discouraged when his weight didn't change after four weeks of macro tracking. However, upon reviewing his progress photos and measurements, we discovered that he had lost two inches from his waist while gaining muscle definition in his arms and chest. This revelation transformed his approach to progress monitoring and reinforced the importance of tracking multiple indicators.

When it comes to fine-tuning your macros, small, systematic adjustments are key. Rather than making dramatic changes, aim to adjust one macro at a time by 5-10% of total calories. This methodical approach helps identify which changes are most effective for your body while maintaining overall dietary balance.

Create a structured monitoring system by:

- Taking progress photos every 2-4 weeks

- Recording measurements monthly

- Keeping a brief daily journal of energy levels and hunger signals

- Tracking workout performance weekly

- Reviewing and adjusting macros every 3-4 weeks

Remember that progress isn't always linear. Your body may respond differently to the same macro distribution at different times due to factors such as stress, sleep quality, hormonal changes, and varying activity levels. This is why regular monitoring and adjustment are crucial for long-term success.

I recommend using a simple tracking template that includes both objective measurements and subjective feedback. This combination provides a more complete picture of your progress and helps identify patterns that might not be apparent from numbers alone.

When making macro adjustments, consider these guidelines:

- Start with carbohydrate adjustments first, as they often have the most immediate impact on energy and performance

- Maintain protein intake during adjustment periods to preserve muscle mass

- Make fat adjustments based on energy levels and hormonal response

- Allow at least 2-3 weeks between significant macro changes to assess their impact properly

One effective strategy I've found is the "macro cycling" approach, where you adjust your macro ratios based on your activity levels and recovery needs. For example, increasing carbohydrates on training days while slightly reducing them on rest days can help optimize both performance and body composition.

During my work with clients, I've observed that the most successful long-term results come from those who view progress monitoring as a learning process rather than a judgment system. Each measurement, whether it shows progress or not, provides valuable information about how your body responds to different macro distributions.

Remember that the goal of monitoring and adjustment isn't to achieve perfection, but to create a sustainable approach that supports your health and fitness goals. Be patient with the process and trust that small, consistent adjustments will lead to significant long-term results.

When you notice plateaus or unexpected changes, use this troubleshooting checklist:

- Review your tracking accuracy

- Assess sleep quality and stress levels

- Check adherence to planned macro targets

- Evaluate hydration status

- Consider recent changes in activity level

By maintaining a systematic approach to progress monitoring and macro adjustment, you'll develop a better understanding of your body's unique needs and responses. This knowledge becomes invaluable as you continue to refine your nutrition strategy for long-term success. As we conclude this chapter on smart tracking strategies, remember that successful macro tracking isn't about achieving perfect precision but developing sustainable systems that work for your lifestyle. Through Tom's journey from stressed-out traveler to confident macro tracker, we've seen how simplifying our approach can lead to better long-term results. The key isn't in weighing every morsel but in building practical habits that last.

We've explored various tracking methods, from high-tech apps to simple hand measurements, each offering unique benefits for different lifestyles. These tools are meant to serve you, not control you. Whether you prefer the precision of digital tracking or the simplicity of visual portion guides, the best method is the one you can maintain consistently.

The strategies we've covered— from basic food logging to advanced meal template creation—form a comprehensive toolkit for your macronutrition journey. Remember that tracking is a skill that develops over time, and it's expected to adjust your approach as your needs and lifestyle change. Start with the basics, focus on consistency over perfection, and gradually refine your system as you become more comfortable with the process.

Moving forward, I encourage you to experiment with different tracking methods to find what resonates with you. Begin with a straightforward change, perhaps using hand measurements for portion control or pre-logging typical meals, and build from there. Remember Tom's transformation - it didn't happen overnight, but through consistent application of manageable strategies.

As you continue your macro-nutrition journey, keep in mind that tracking is just one piece of the puzzle. In the next chapter, we'll explore how to personalize your macro ratios based on your unique body type and goals, building upon the tracking foundation we've established here. The tools and techniques you've learned will serve as the framework for making informed adjustments to your nutrition plan.

Your success in macro tracking doesn't depend on following a perfect system but on finding an approach that fits seamlessly into your life while supporting your health and fitness goals. Trust in the process, stay consistent with your chosen method, and remember that sustainable progress comes from practical, maintainable habits rather than temporary perfection.

Chapter 8

Sustainable Success: Making Macro Nutrition a Lifestyle

In today's digital age, tracking your nutrition has never been more accessible, yet many people feel overwhelmed by the abundance of options and information available. The key to successful macro tracking isn't finding the perfect app or system, but instead discovering the method that seamlessly integrates into your daily routine while providing the insights you need to reach your goals. The journey to finding your ideal tracking method is deeply personal, much like discovering the perfect workout routine or morning ritual that resonates with your lifestyle. While some individuals thrive with detailed digital tracking, others prefer more straightforward methods, such as photo logging or template-based approaches. The key lies in identifying a system that provides the insights you need without becoming a source of stress or obsession.

I've seen firsthand how the right tracking strategy can transform someone's nutrition journey. During a nutrition workshop I was leading, I met a client named Lisa who was struggling with macro tracking. She had downloaded multiple tracking apps but found herself spending hours each day weighing food, logging entries, and second-guessing her measurements. Her tracking habits were becoming obsessive, and she was losing the joy of eating. Together, we developed a simplified approach that utilizes meal templates and photo logging for regular meals, reserving detailed tracking for special occasions or new events. We created a system where she pre-logged her common breakfast and lunch options, then focused more attention on dinner variations. Within a month, Lisa reported spending just 5-10 minutes daily on tracking while maintaining consistent progress toward her goals. She rediscovered the pleasure of cooking and eating with her family, proving that effective tracking doesn't require constant digital input or perfect precision. Her transformation from overwhelmed to empowered perfectly illustrates how finding the right balance in monitoring can make all the difference in sustaining healthy habits.

In this chapter, we'll explore various tracking methods and tools, ranging from sophisticated apps to simple journal techniques, to help you discover which approach aligns best with your personality and goals. You'll learn practical strategies for maintaining accuracy without becoming overly rigid and develop skills for tracking in challenging situations, such as dining out or traveling. Most importantly, you'll learn how to create a sustainable tracking system that enhances, rather than dominates, your relationship with food.

Whether you're new to macro tracking or seeking to refine your current approach, the techniques and strategies in this chapter will help you develop a practical and sustainable system tailored to your unique lifestyle. Remember, the goal isn't perfect adherence to numbers, but instead creating awareness and understanding that supports your long-term nutrition success.

Building Sustainable Habits: From Knowledge to Lifestyle Integration

Transforming nutrition knowledge into sustainable habits requires more than just understanding macros - it demands a systematic approach to behavior change. The journey from knowing what to do to consistently doing it is where many people struggle. However, by breaking down this transformation into manageable steps and creating supportive systems, you can build lasting habits that make macro-nutrition feel as natural as brushing your teeth.

One of the most effective strategies I've found for habit formation is what I call the "anchor method." This involves attaching new nutrition habits to existing daily routines. For instance, if you already have a morning coffee routine, use this time to plan your macro goals for the day. If you regularly prep your work clothes the night before, pair this with preparing the next day's lunch. These small but consistent actions create powerful habit chains that support your nutrition goals.

I recall working with a client named Marcus, who struggled to maintain a consistent protein intake despite understanding its importance. Instead of overwhelming him with complex tracking requirements, we started with a straightforward habit: adding a protein source to his existing breakfast routine. Once this became automatic, we gradually built upon this foundation, adding more structured macro planning throughout his day. Within three months, what started as a single habit had evolved into a comprehensive but manageable nutrition system.

The key to forming sustainable habits lies in making small, incremental changes rather than attempting dramatic overhauls. Start by identifying one or two key areas where improved macro-nutrition would make the most significant impact on your goals. Perhaps it's ensuring adequate protein at each meal or incorporating more fiber-rich carbohydrates into your diet. Focus on mastering these fundamental habits before adding more complexity.

Environmental design plays a crucial role in habit sustainability. Your surroundings should support, not sabotage, your nutrition goals. This might involve reorganizing your kitchen to make macro-friendly foods more accessible, batch-preparing protein sources for easy meal assembly, or keeping healthy snacks visible and within easy reach. The easier you make it to follow your macro targets, the more likely you are to maintain them in the long term.

Another essential aspect of habit formation is developing response strategies for everyday challenges. Life inevitably throws curveballs - busy workdays, social events, travel - but having pre-planned solutions helps maintain consistency. Create simple decision trees for different situations: if the office provides lunch, choose protein first and fill half your plate with vegetables. If dining out, review the menu ahead of time and identify macro-friendly options.

Tracking progress is vital, but it's essential to focus on behavioral metrics rather than just numerical data. Instead of obsessing over hitting exact macro targets, celebrate consistency in habits like meal preparation, grocery shopping, and mindful eating. These foundational behaviors ultimately lead to better adherence to your macro goals while fostering a healthier relationship with food.

Remember that setbacks are a normal part of forming a habit. Rather than viewing them as failures, treat them as opportunities for learning. Each challenge provides valuable insights into your triggers, obstacles, and areas that require additional support or strategic adjustments. This growth mindset helps maintain momentum even when perfect adherence isn't possible.

As you progress in your macro-nutrition journey, periodically reassess and refine your habits. What worked during one life phase might need adjustment during another. The goal isn't to create rigid rules, but to develop flexible and adaptable systems that evolve with your changing needs while maintaining core nutritional principles.

Ultimately, sustainable success in macro-nutrition comes from transforming knowledge into intuitive daily practices. By focusing on progressive habit building, environmental design, and consistent but flexible systems, you can create a sustainable approach to nutrition that supports your goals without dominating your life. Remember, it's not about being perfect - it's about being consistent enough to see results while maintaining balance and enjoyment in your relationship with food.

Mindset Shifts: Moving Beyond the Diet Mentality

One of the most significant challenges in developing a healthy relationship with macro-nutrition isn't mastering the numbers or understanding the science - it's shifting away from the restrictive mindset that often accompanies traditional dieting. The diet mentality, characterized by rigid rules, all-or-nothing thinking, and moral judgments about food choices, can sabotage even the most well-planned nutrition strategy. Moving beyond this mindset requires a fundamental shift in how we think about food, nutrition, and our relationship with eating.

I witnessed this transformation firsthand while working with a client named Claire, who came to me after years of cycling through various restrictive diets. She had internalized so many rules about 'good' and 'bad' foods that even the thought of eating carbohydrates triggered anxiety. Together, we worked on reframing her approach to nutrition, focusing on understanding macronutrients as tools for fueling her body rather than enemies to be avoided. Instead of viewing foods as 'forbidden' or 'allowed,' we explored how different combinations of macronutrients could support her energy levels, workout performance, and overall well-being.

The first step in moving beyond the diet mentality is recognizing that macro-nutrition isn't about restriction - it's about understanding and optimizing your food choices to support your goals. This means letting go of perfectionist tendencies and embracing flexibility. A balanced macro approach allows for all foods in moderation, focusing on the overall pattern of eating rather than individual food choices.

One practical strategy for shifting your mindset is to start thinking in terms of additions rather than restrictions. Instead of focusing on foods to eliminate, consider adding nutritious options to your meals. For example, rather than viewing a meal as 'lacking protein,' think about creative ways to incorporate protein-rich foods you enjoy. This subtle shift from restriction to enhancement can have a profound impact on your relationship with food and nutrition.

Another crucial aspect of moving beyond the diet mentality is developing trust in your body's signals while maintaining awareness of your macro goals. This means learning to balance hunger and fullness cues with nutritional knowledge. For instance, if you're craving carbohydrates after an intense workout, this might be your body's way of signaling its need for replenishment. Instead of fighting these signals, work on understanding them and responding with balanced choices that align with your macro targets.

Let go of the concept of 'perfect' eating days. In macro-nutrition, consistency over time matters more than day-to-day precision. On some days, you may be slightly over your carbohydrate target but under your protein target; this is normal. What matters is your overall pattern of eating and your ability to maintain a balanced approach most of the time.

Practice self-compassion when facing challenges or setbacks. If you overeat at a social event or miss your macro targets during a stressful week, treat these situations as learning opportunities rather than failures. Ask yourself what you can learn from the experience and how you might handle similar situations in the future, rather than falling into the cycle of guilt and restriction that characterizes the diet mentality.

Develop a flexible approach to special occasions and social events. Instead of viewing these situations as threats to your nutrition goals, see them as opportunities to practice balance and moderation. This might mean adjusting your macros before or after an event, or simply accepting that some days will look different than others without trying to compensate through restriction.

Remember that your adherence to macro targets or any other nutrition metrics doesn't determine your worth. While tracking macros can be a valuable tool for reaching health and fitness goals, it shouldn't become a source of stress or anxiety. If you find yourself becoming overly focused on numbers or feeling guilty about food choices, take a step back and reassess your approach.

The journey from a diet mentality to a balanced, sustainable approach to macro-nutrition is ongoing. It requires patience, practice, and consistent reinforcement of healthy thought patterns. Focus on progress over perfection, and celebrate the small victories along the way - like choosing foods based on how they make you feel rather than arbitrary rules, or maintaining consistent energy levels throughout the day through balanced macro intake.

By shifting away from the diet mentality, you create space for a more sustainable, enjoyable approach to nutrition. This mindset shift enables you to utilize macro-nutrition as a tool for supporting your health and fitness goals while fostering a positive relationship with food and eating. Remember, the goal isn't to control food - it's to understand and work with it in a way that enhances your life rather than restricting it.

Adapting Your Macro Approach Through Life Changes

Life is a journey of constant change, and your macro-nutrition approach needs to evolve alongside these transitions. Whether you're experiencing changes in your activity level, entering a new life phase, or adapting to different schedules, maintaining optimal nutrition requires thoughtful adjustments to your macro intake. Understanding how to adjust your approach while keeping your core nutrition principles is key to long-term success.

One of the most significant transitions I've guided clients through is pregnancy and postpartum nutrition. I worked with Sarah, a dedicated runner who discovered she was pregnant shortly after mastering her macro balance for performance. Together, we adjusted her macro approach to support her changing needs - gradually increasing protein intake to support fetal development, adjusting carbohydrates to manage morning sickness, and ensuring adequate healthy fats for hormonal balance. After delivery, we created a new plan that supported her recovery and breastfeeding needs while gradually working toward her return to running.

Career changes can also significantly impact your macro needs. When transitioning from an active job to a desk-based role, or vice versa, your energy requirements and macro distribution need adjustment. Consider the case of Michael, who moved from construction work to an office position. His daily energy expenditure decreased significantly, necessitating adjustments to his carbohydrate intake while maintaining protein levels to preserve muscle mass. We developed strategies for incorporating movement throughout his workday and adjusted meal timing to prevent the afternoon energy crashes common with sedentary work.

Seasonal changes and travel can also necessitate macro adjustments. During warmer months, you might notice increased fluid needs and changes in appetite. Winter often brings cravings for heartier meals and different energy requirements. Rather than fighting these natural variations, work with them by adjusting your macro distribution while maintaining overall balanced nutrition. For example, you might increase your intake of hydrating fruits and vegetables in summer while focusing on warming, nutrient-dense foods in winter.

Stress and sleep patterns significantly influence how your body processes and utilizes macronutrients. During high-stress periods, your body may require additional protein and complex carbohydrates to maintain energy levels and support recovery. Pay attention to how your body responds to different macro ratios during these times, and don't hesitate to make adjustments that support your well-being.

Training cycles and fitness goals naturally evolve, necessitating corresponding adjustments to your macro approach. Whether you're transitioning from a building phase to a cutting phase or shifting from endurance training to a focus on strength, your macro needs will vary. The key is making gradual adjustments while monitoring your body's response and performance markers.

Age-related changes also influence macro requirements. As metabolism naturally shifts with age, protein needs often increase while carbohydrate tolerance may decrease. Focus on high-quality protein sources and nutrient-dense carbohydrates, adjusting portions and timing to match your changing energy levels. Regular reassessment of your macro needs helps ensure that your nutrition continues to support your health goals as you age.

When adapting your macro approach, remember that changes should be gradual and systematic. Start with minor adjustments of 5-10% in any macro category and monitor your response over 2-3 weeks before making further modifications. Pay attention to energy levels, hunger cues, sleep quality, and performance markers to guide your adjustments.

Maintaining flexibility in your macro approach doesn't mean abandoning structure entirely. Develop systems that can adapt to various scenarios while maintaining your core nutritional principles. For instance, develop a set of go-to meals that can be easily modified to meet different macro needs, or establish basic guidelines for adjusting portions based on activity level and energy requirements.

Remember that life changes often bring emotional and psychological challenges that can impact your relationship with food. During major transitions, focus first on maintaining consistent, balanced nutrition rather than adhering perfectly to macros. As you adjust to new circumstances, gradually refine your approach to optimize your macro intake while respecting your body's changing needs.

The ability to adapt your macro approach to life's changes is ultimately what makes it sustainable in the long term. By developing this flexibility while maintaining your fundamental nutrition principles, you create a resilient foundation that can support you through any transition. Stay mindful of your body's signals, be patient with the adjustment process, and remember that evolution in your nutrition approach is not only expected but necessary for continued progress and well-being.

Creating Support Systems and Environmental Success Factors

Creating a supportive environment and building reliable support systems are crucial elements for long-term success in your macro-nutrition journey. Just as a garden needs the right conditions to flourish, your nutrition habits thrive best when surrounded by positive influences and practical support structures. Understanding how to shape your environment and build meaningful support networks can make the difference between temporary progress and lasting change.

I've seen the power of environmental design firsthand while working with a client named Jamie, who struggled to maintain consistent macro targets despite having extensive knowledge of nutrition. Her kitchen was organized chaotically, with healthy options hidden behind processed snacks, and her meal prep attempts often failed due to poor planning. Together, we restructured her environment, starting with a kitchen reorganization that placed macro-friendly foods at eye level and created dedicated prep stations for efficient meal assembly. Within weeks, she reported that making nutritious choices had become significantly easier simply because her environment supported her goals.

Your physical environment plays a crucial role in your nutrition success. Begin by conducting an environmental audit of your home, workplace, and other areas where you frequently make food choices. Look for opportunities to make healthy choices more convenient and less nutritious options less accessible. This might mean keeping protein-rich snacks in your desk drawer, storing cut vegetables at eye level in your refrigerator, or setting up a dedicated meal prep station in your kitchen.

Creating systems that reduce decision fatigue is another vital aspect of environmental design. Consider implementing strategies like weekly grocery lists organized by store layout, standardized meal prep routines, and pre-portioned snack containers. These systems make it easier to maintain consistent macro intake without requiring constant willpower or decision-making.

Building a strong support network is equally essential for sustainable success. This network can include family members, friends, workout partners, or nutrition professionals who understand and support your goals. Be selective about who you share your journey with - seek out people who offer encouragement and practical support rather than judgment or negativity.

Technology can also serve as a valuable support system when used mindfully. Consider joining online communities focused on macro-nutrition, using meal planning apps that align with your goals, or following social media accounts that provide reliable nutrition information and inspiration. However, be cautious when using sources that promote extreme approaches or unrealistic expectations.

One effective strategy for building support systems is creating accountability partnerships. Find someone with similar goals and establish regular check-ins to share progress, challenges, and solutions. These partnerships work best when focused on behavior-based goals, rather than just numbers—for example, completing weekly meal prep sessions or trying new macro-friendly recipes.

Your social environment has a significant impact on your nutrition habits. Work on developing strategies for maintaining your macro goals in different social situations. This might include having conversations with family members about your nutrition goals, suggesting macro-friendly restaurants for social gatherings, or learning to navigate workplace food environments effectively.

Remember that support systems need regular maintenance and updating. As your goals evolve and life circumstances change, your support needs may shift. Regularly assess what's working and what isn't, and don't hesitate to make adjustments to your support network or environmental setup as needed.

Professional support can also play a valuable role in your macro-nutrition journey. Consider working with a qualified nutrition professional who can provide personalized guidance, troubleshoot challenges, and help you develop effective strategies for your specific situation. This investment in professional support often pays dividends in faster progress and fewer setbacks.

Creating success factors in your environment extends beyond food-related elements. Consider how sleep quality, stress management, and daily routines impact your ability to maintain consistent nutrition habits. Design your environment to support these foundational factors, such as creating a relaxing bedtime routine or setting up a dedicated home workout space.

The key to achieving sustainable environmental success lies in making these factors personal and practical for your lifestyle. What works for someone else might not work for you, and that's okay. Focus on creating systems and support structures that align with your preferences, schedule, and goals while remaining flexible enough to adapt as needed.

Remember that building effective support systems and environmental success factors is an ongoing process. Start with small, manageable changes and gradually build upon them as they become habitual. Celebrate the progress you make along the way, and use challenges as opportunities to refine and strengthen your support structures. With the right environment and support network in place, maintaining your macronutrient goals becomes significantly more achievable and sustainable in the long term.

Long-term Progress Monitoring and Habit Maintenance

Monitoring your progress and maintaining healthy habits over the long term requires a balanced approach that combines consistent tracking with flexibility. While the initial excitement of starting a new nutrition journey can fuel motivation, sustaining these practices requires developing systems that work with your lifestyle rather than against it. The key lies in finding the right balance between awareness and obsession, using data to inform your choices while maintaining a healthy relationship with food.

One of the most effective strategies I've found for long-term monitoring is what I call the "checkpoint method." Rather than tracking every detail daily, establish regular intervals—perhaps weekly or monthly—for reviewing your progress more comprehensively. During these checkpoints, assess not only your macro adherence but also other important markers, such as energy levels, sleep quality, and performance in your daily activities. This broader view helps maintain perspective and prevents the tunnel vision that often comes with focusing solely on numbers.

I worked with a client named Teresa who initially struggled with maintaining consistent tracking habits. She would meticulously log everything for a few weeks, then become overwhelmed and abandon tracking altogether. Together, we developed a simplified system that focused on key meals and specific days of the week rather than requiring constant logging. She tracked her breakfast and dinner macros Monday through Thursday, then used general guidelines for other meals and weekend days. This balanced approach allowed her to maintain awareness of her nutrition while preventing burnout.

When it comes to maintaining habits, the concept of the "minimum effective dose" proves invaluable. Identify the core habits that yield the most significant results for your goals, and focus on maintaining these consistently. For many people, this may include practices such as weekly meal prep, protein-first meal planning, or regular grocery shopping routines. By prioritizing these fundamental habits, you create a strong foundation that can weather life's inevitable disruptions.

Progress monitoring should extend beyond just tracking macros and weight changes. Consider keeping a simple journal to note your energy levels, workout performance, sleep quality, and overall well-being. These subjective markers often provide valuable insights into how well your current macro balance is serving your needs. They can also help identify patterns and triggers that affect your nutrition habits, allowing for more targeted adjustments when needed.

Technology can be a valuable ally in long-term monitoring, but it's essential to use it mindfully. While tracking apps offer convenience, they shouldn't become a source of stress or obsession. Consider utilizing features such as meal templates and quick-logging options to streamline the process. Some people find that taking photos of their meals provides sufficient accountability, as it is less time-consuming than detailed tracking.

Regular environmental audits play a crucial role in maintaining habits. Every few months, assess your food environment, meal prep systems, and support structures. Are your kitchen and workspace organized to support your nutrition goals? Do you have reliable backup plans for busy days? These periodic reviews help identify areas where your systems might need updating or reinforcement.

One often-overlooked aspect of long-term success is the ability to adapt your monitoring strategies across different life phases. What works during a period of strict training might not be sustainable during busier or more stressful times. Develop different levels of tracking intensity that you can shift between as needed, while maintaining core habits that support your nutrition goals.

Celebrate consistency over perfection in your long-term journey. Rather than focusing on perfect macro adherence, acknowledge the maintenance of key habits and the ability to return to them after disruptions. This might mean recognizing that you've maintained your weekly meal prep routine for three months straight, or that you've consistently hit your protein targets despite a challenging work schedule.

Remember that sustainable progress often follows a non-linear path. There will be periods of strict adherence and times when you need more flexibility. The key is maintaining awareness of these natural cycles and adjusting your monitoring approach accordingly. This may involve increasing tracking detail during focused training phases and reducing it during maintenance periods.

Establish regular check-ins with yourself or a nutrition professional to review your progress and adjust your approach as needed. These reviews should examine both quantitative measures (such as macro adherence and changes in body composition) and qualitative factors (such as energy levels and satisfaction with the current routine). Utilize these insights to make informed adjustments to your nutrition strategy while maintaining focus on your long-term goals.

Ultimately, successful long-term progress monitoring and habit maintenance come from finding the sweet spot between structure and flexibility. It's about developing systems that provide enough accountability to keep you on track while being sustainable enough to maintain over time. Remember that the goal isn't perfect tracking or adherence, but relatively consistent progress toward your health and fitness objectives while maintaining a healthy relationship with food and nutrition. As we conclude this chapter on innovative tracking strategies, it's essential to remember that the most effective tracking method is one you can maintain consistently over time. Through the examples and techniques we've explored, it's clear that successful macro tracking isn't about finding the perfect system, but instead discovering an approach that integrates seamlessly into your lifestyle while providing the insights needed to reach your goals.

We've seen how Lisa transformed her relationship with tracking from an obsessive, time-consuming process into a streamlined system that took just minutes per day. Her story reminds us that effectiveness doesn't always correlate with complexity - sometimes, the most straightforward approaches yield the best results. The key strategies we've covered, from meal templating to photo logging, offer various ways to maintain macro awareness without letting tracking dominate your life.

The journey to finding your ideal tracking method is deeply personal. Whether you choose digital apps, paper journals, or a combination of techniques, what matters most is that your chosen system supports rather than hinders your relationship with food. Remember that tracking is a tool to enhance your nutrition journey, not a measure of your worth or success.

As you move forward, experiment with different tracking approaches we've discussed to find what resonates best with your lifestyle. Begin with one method and allow yourself time to adapt before making any adjustments. Pay attention to how different tracking strategies affect not just your macro adherence but also your overall relationship with food and eating habits.

Most importantly, remember that tracking methods can and should evolve with you. What works during one phase of your life might need adjustment during another. The flexibility to adapt your tracking approach while maintaining core principles is what makes it sustainable in the long term.

Your success in macro-nutrition isn't measured by the precision of your tracking but by your ability to maintain consistent, healthy habits that support your goals while enjoying the journey along the way.

Conclusion

As we reach the end of our macro-nutrition journey together, I'm reminded of the transformative power of understanding and applying these fundamental principles of nutrition. Throughout this book, we've explored how macronutrients serve as the building blocks of a healthy, sustainable approach to eating. We've learned that successful nutrition isn't about following rigid rules or achieving perfect numbers, but rather about developing an informed, flexible approach that adapts to your unique needs and lifestyle.

I've shared stories from my journey and those of my clients, demonstrating how macro-nutrition can be adapted to various life situations, from busy professionals managing hectic schedules to athletes pursuing performance goals. Each story reinforces a crucial truth: there is no one-size-fits-all approach to nutrition. Your path to success lies in understanding the principles we've covered and adapting them to fit your individual needs, preferences, and goals.

As you move forward with your macro-nutrition journey, keep these key principles in mind: macronutrients are tools for better health, not restrictions to limit your life. Tracking should inform your choices, not control them. And most importantly, your nutrition approach should enhance your life, not complicate it.

The strategies, tools, and knowledge you've gained from this book provide a foundation for long-term success. Whether your goal is weight management, improved athletic performance, or simply better overall health, the principles of macro-nutrition can help you achieve it. Remember that progress isn't always linear, and perfection isn't the goal – consistency and sustainability are what matter most.

I encourage you to start implementing these concepts gradually, focusing on one change at a time. Begin with understanding your current eating patterns, then slowly adjust your macro intake to better align with your goals. Use the tracking methods that work best for you, whether that's detailed app logging or simple portion awareness. Most importantly, be patient with yourself as you develop these new habits.

Your journey with macro-nutrition doesn't end with the last page of this book. Consider this the beginning of a new chapter in your relationship with food – one based on knowledge, awareness, and balanced choices. The principles you've learned here will continue to serve you as your goals and circumstances evolve.

Thank you for allowing me to be part of your nutrition journey. Remember, every step forward, no matter how small, is progress toward your goals. Trust in the process, stay consistent with the basics, and keep adjusting your approach as needed. Here's to your continued success in mastering macro-nutrition and creating a sustainable, healthy relationship with food that will serve you for years to come.

And finally, thank you for choosing my book to help on your wellness journey. If you have enjoyed this book, I'd be so grateful if you could leave a review on Amazon. Your feedback will help me, and also help others discover and enjoy my books.

All the best in your health and wellness journey, Amelia xx

Other books by Amelia Evans

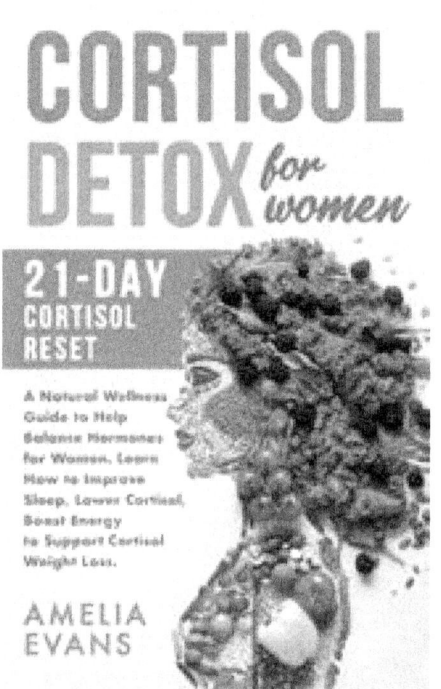

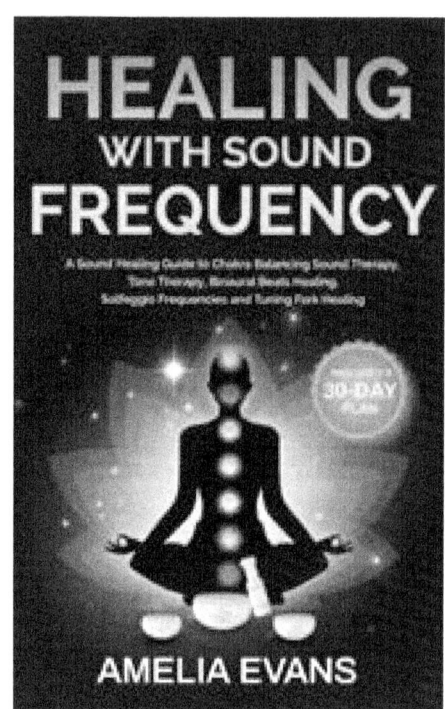

Bibliography

American College of Sports Medicine. (2021). ACSM's Guidelines for Exercise Testing and Prescription. Wolters Kluwer.

Burke, L. M., & Deakin, V. (2015). Clinical Sports Nutrition (5th ed.). McGraw-Hill Education.

Helms, E. R., Aragon, A. A., & Fitschen, P. J. (2014). Evidence-based recommendations for natural bodybuilding contest preparation: nutrition and supplementation. Journal of the International Society of Sports Nutrition, 11(1), 20.

Jäger, R., Kerksick, C. M., Campbell, B. I., et al. (2017). International Society of Sports Nutrition Position Stand: protein and exercise. Journal of the International Society of Sports Nutrition, 14, 20.

Kerksick, C. M., Wilborn, C. D., Roberts, M. D., et al. (2018). ISSN exercise & sports nutrition review update: research & recommendations. Journal of the International Society of Sports Nutrition, 15(1), 38.

Maughan, R. J. (Ed.). (2014). Sports Nutrition (The Encyclopaedia of Sports Medicine Book 19). Wiley-Blackwell.

Phillips, S. M., & Van Loon, L. J. (2011). Dietary protein for athletes: from requirements to optimum adaptation. Journal of Sports Sciences, 29(sup1), S29-S38.

Stoppani, J. (2013). Encyclopedia of Muscle & Strength (2nd ed.). Human Kinetics.

Thomas, D. T., Erdman, K. A., & Burke, L. M. (2016). Position of the Academy of Nutrition and Dietetics, Dietitians of Canada, and the American College of Sports Medicine: Nutrition and Athletic Performance. Journal of the Academy of Nutrition and Dietetics, 116(3), 501-528.

Tipton, K. D., & Wolfe, R. R. (2004). Protein and amino acids for athletes. Journal of Sports Sciences, 22(1), 65-79.

Printed in Dunstable, United Kingdom

66508173R00097